Table for One

Table for One

Perfectly portioned meals for the single cook

Camille Funk

CFI

Springville, Utah

ISBN 13: 978-1-59955-432-7

Published by CFI, an imprint of Cedar Fort, Inc., 2373 W. 700 S., Springville, UT 84663
Distributed by Cedar Fort, Inc., www.cedarfort.com

Library of Congress Cataloging-in-Publication Data

Funk, Camille.
Table for one / Camille Funk.
p. cm.
Includes index.
ISBN 978-1-59955-432-7
1. Cookery for one. I. Title.

TX652.F86 2010
641.5'61--dc22

2010012375

Cover and page design by Tanya Quinlan
Cover design © 2010 by Lyle Mortimer
Edited by Kimiko Christensen Hammari

Printed in China

10 9 8 7 6 5 4 3 2 1

To my taste-testing roommates
Lindsey Andersen and Lindsey Sellers
and my loving family.

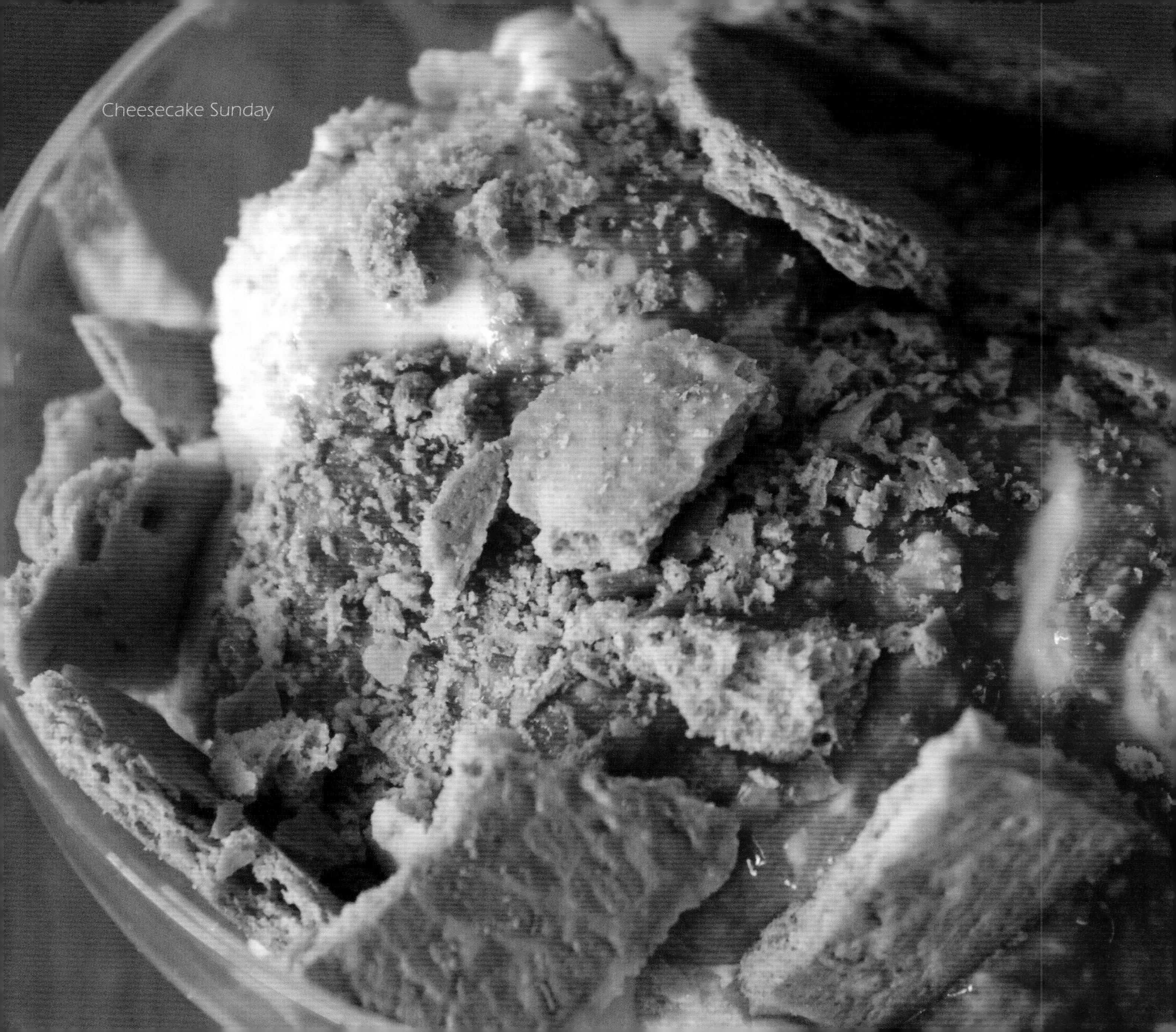
Cheesecake Sunday

Table of Contents

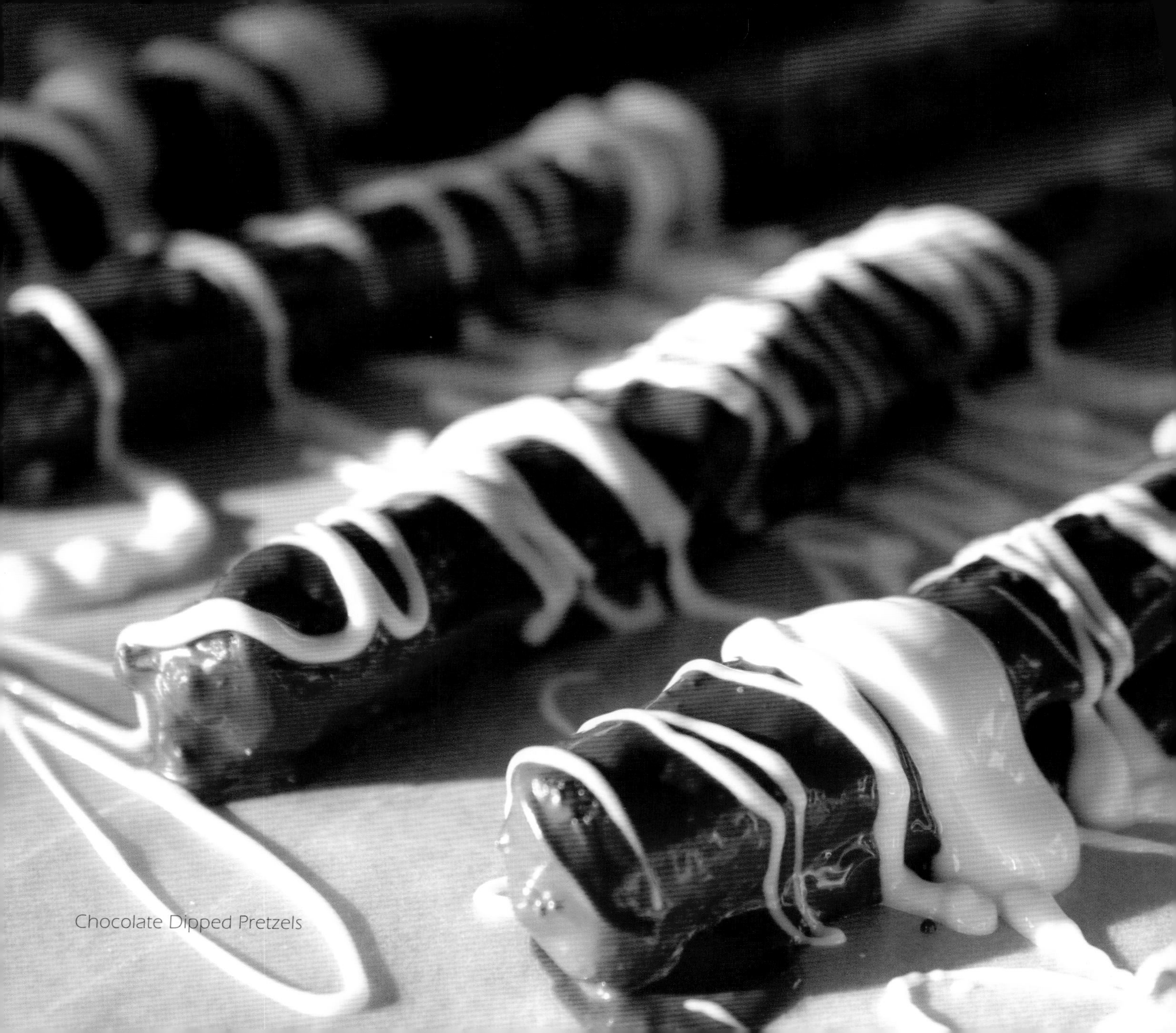

Chocolate Dipped Pretzels

Introduction

Most of us know from experience that cooking for one takes some adjustment. When I was a freshman in college, I would make my mother's recipes and either end up eating for much more than just one, or having the same leftovers for a week straight. While the dish was tasty, I was bored with the lack of variety.

Over the years, I have found that I can have all the same types of dishes I love and adore, modified for my lifestyle. In cooking my mother's recipes, I learned some valuable lessons about how to prepare different types of food and how to make adjustments as needed for my budget and lifestyle. I hope to pass on some of these lessons and share what I have learned about food preparation and cooking tips.

Food Preparation

Herbs

One of the biggest potential wastes for me as a single woman was purchasing herbs. Usually I only needed 1 teaspoon or one stem to complete my meal, and since herbs are sold in fairly large quantities, the herb would sit in the fridge and rot. The next time I needed the herb, it was no longer edible, and I had to purchase another package of herbs, which had the same fate. However, I have a few suggestions to help prevent this waste.

1. **Herb Garden**—Purchase a medium-sized pot for plants and 3–4 of the herbs you use the most. Plant and water them as needed, and you will rarely need to purchase more than

you grow. (Recommended herbs are basil, mint, parsley, rosemary, sage, and cilantro.)

2. **Ingredient Index**—Realizing an herb garden may not be an option for everyone, I can recommend one more thing: the ingredient index at the end of this book. I have put all perishable items (including herbs) in bold face throughout this cookbook, and have included an index of perishable ingredients for you to reference. The ingredient index lists all recipes that include that perishable ingredient, so you can plan your meals around those items and get the maximum use out of your dollar.

Measurements

One of the most important things in cooking for one is making sure your measurements are just right, especially since they are a bit unusual at times. That's why I have come to love my food scale. When I can measure out portions that I don't usually have a preset spoon or cup for, I can ensure that I get just the right amount.

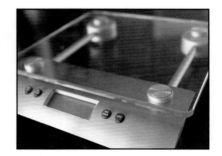

Pantry Stocking

The next thing we need to talk about is how to stock your pantry. It is useful to have some of the basics used in several dishes, such as:

- **Diced garlic cloves** (in a jar)—This has been one of my best finds. The garlic is already diced and put into a jar to ensure long-lasting preservation. This item will need to be refrigerated.
- **Spices/Dried herbs**—Purchasing spices all at once can be expensive, so I made a goal

of purchasing a new dried herb or spice each time I went to the grocery store, until I had a solid base.

- **Bouillon cubes**—I use these as a substitute if recipes call for chicken (or beef) broth/stock and I don't have a can on hand. They are great to have handy when you can't quite make it to the store.
- **Sugar**—Three basic types of sugar will be used in this cookbook: white granulated sugar, brown sugar, and confectioners' (powdered) sugar.
- **Flour**—Two types of flour are used in this cookbook: regular (bleached or unbleached) all-purpose flour (referred to as flour) and cake flour. If you would like to be a bit more healthy, you are welcome to switch the all-purpose flour to wheat flour.
- **Oils**—This cookbook calls for a few types of oil: extra virgin olive oil (which is referred to as olive oil), sesame seed oil, and vegetable oil. Because of their long shelf life, it is great to purchase all three so that you have them on hand.
- **Vinegars**—This cookbook uses five basic types of vinegars: red wine vinegar, white wine vinegar, rice vinegar, cider vinegar, and white distilled vinegar. Each present a different flavor and dimension to a dish.

Storage

The first issue to tackle is how to buy and store items that come in bulk (or exceed the amount you need for one meal). The biggest concern is perishable items such as meat and fruits and vegetables. The key is in using Ziploc bags and small Tupperware containers. These baggies and containers are essential when cooking for one. They will keep meat and produce fresh, allowing you to stretch your dollar. Let's talk more about how to store produce, meat, and leftovers.

Produce

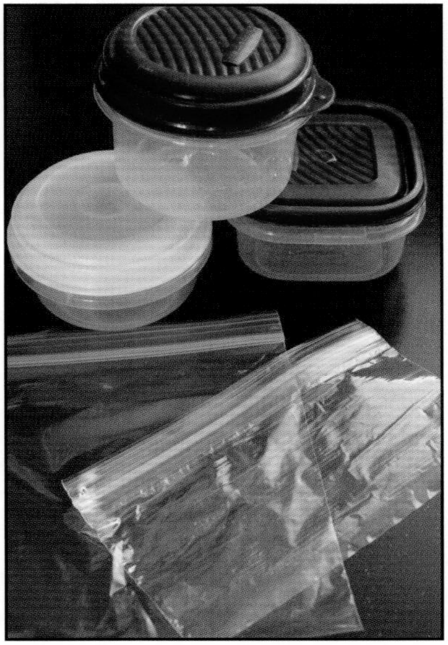

Grapes are my favorite fruit, but you don't have the option of purchasing just a handful when you're at the grocery store. The key, then, lies in the way you store them. The snack-sized Ziploc baggies are very useful. I typically wash and split up my grapes into adequate serving sizes. When I leave for work, I grab a baggie on the way out the door for a snack. Or I can grab a baggie from the fridge when I need a simple side dish to complete a meal.

Again, the key here is to take time right after you purchase produce to wash it, prepare it, split it up into proper serving sizes, and place it in storable Ziploc baggies. This will help you make the produce last in serving sizes for one.

Meat

Meat is tricky, mostly because unless you purchase it from the butcher's counter (which I highly recommend), you rarely get an amount fit for only one meal. But this isn't so bad. Again, the trick is coming home from the supermarket and taking time to portion out your meat into appropriate serving sizes and put it in Ziploc bags. For instance, if I were to purchase three chicken breasts, I would put each one in its own Ziploc bag. Then I would label the meat and include the date I purchased it. The beauty of placing the meat into baggies is that you can reach into the freezer and grab a chicken breast for your meal and use the others when you have another meal that requires them. Now you don't have to feel like you have to cook all the meat at the same time. Additionally, this assists in keeping all the meat fresh, because if you are defrosting all of the meat but only intend to use one chicken breast, you are potentially ruining the rest of the meat with multiple defrosting sessions.

Ingredient Leftovers

I have found that you can't get out of buying certain items en masse—for instance, stewed tomatoes. Even though you can buy a small can, sometimes all you need is a tablespoon or two. In this case, small Tupperware containers do a great job of preserving extra ingredients to use in other recipes. I highly recommend having these small containers on hand, because they will free up space in your fridge. Also, it is good to label what you are storing. You can do this by placing masking tape on the container and writing the name of the product and date. Sometimes it is hard to tell the difference between cream of chicken soup and coconut milk, and that label will help you know at a quick glance what you need to purchase more of at the store.

Cooking Tips

Grill

I highly recommend using a small George Foreman grill, which you can buy for twenty to thirty dollars. This works perfectly for the small portions you will be cooking and will prevent you from having to fire up a large grill.

Baking Dishes

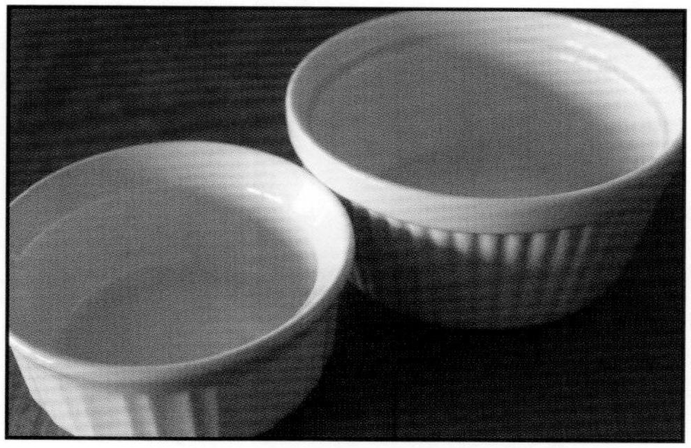

The best addition to the kitchen for someone cooking for one is ramekin dishes. These dishes are oven proof and small enough to hold the small portion of one meal. In this cookbook I use two different dish sizes: a small ramekin (about 3 inches in diameter) and a medium ramekin (about 5 inches in diameter). I highly recommend purchasing these baking dishes. You'll notice the difference in your meals; the flavor will be more concentrated.

Meat Thermometer

A thermometer is essential when cooking with meat. Each oven works a bit differently, but if you know the desired temperature needed to thoroughly cook the meat, you will never go wrong.

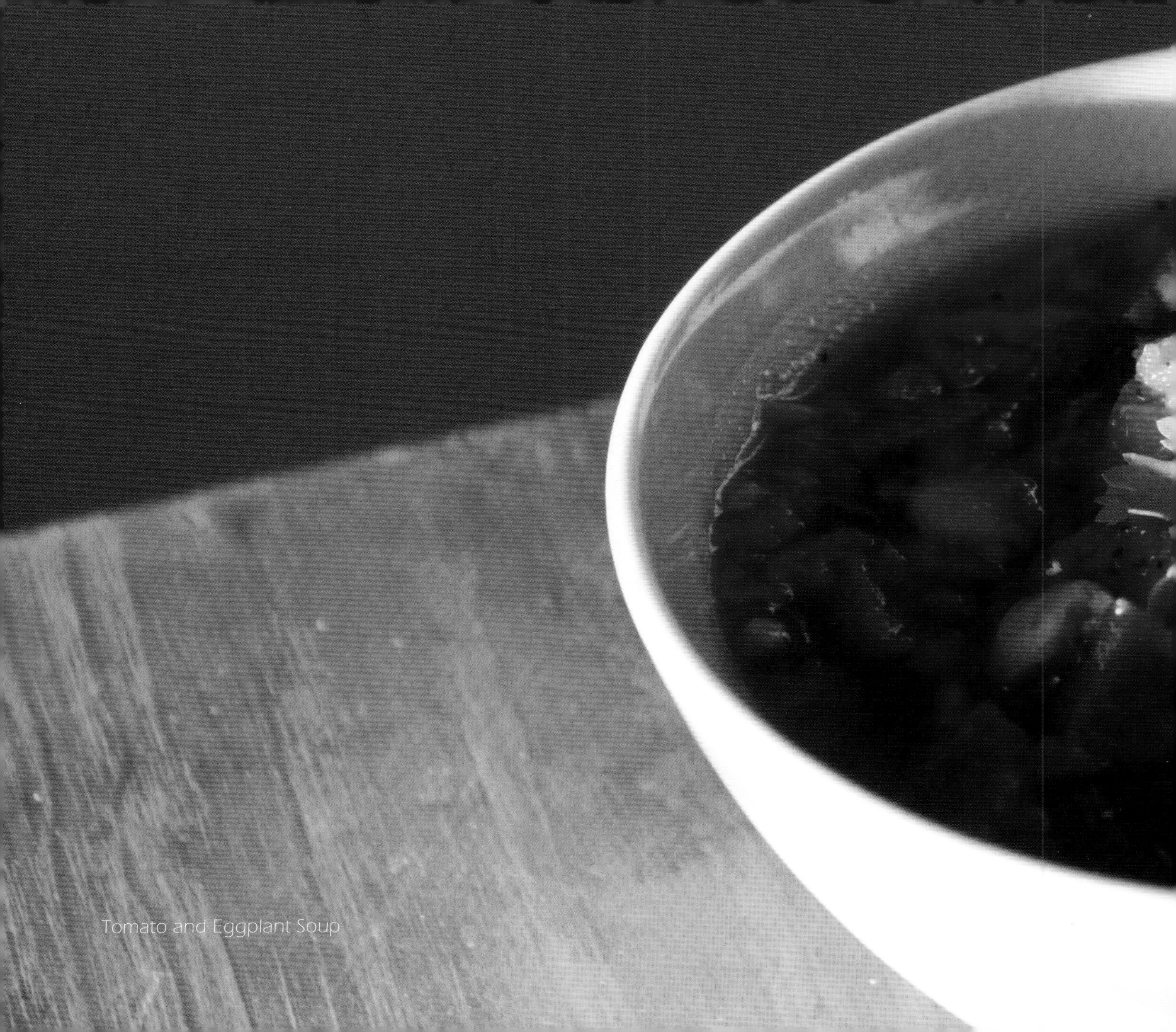

Tomato and Eggplant Soup

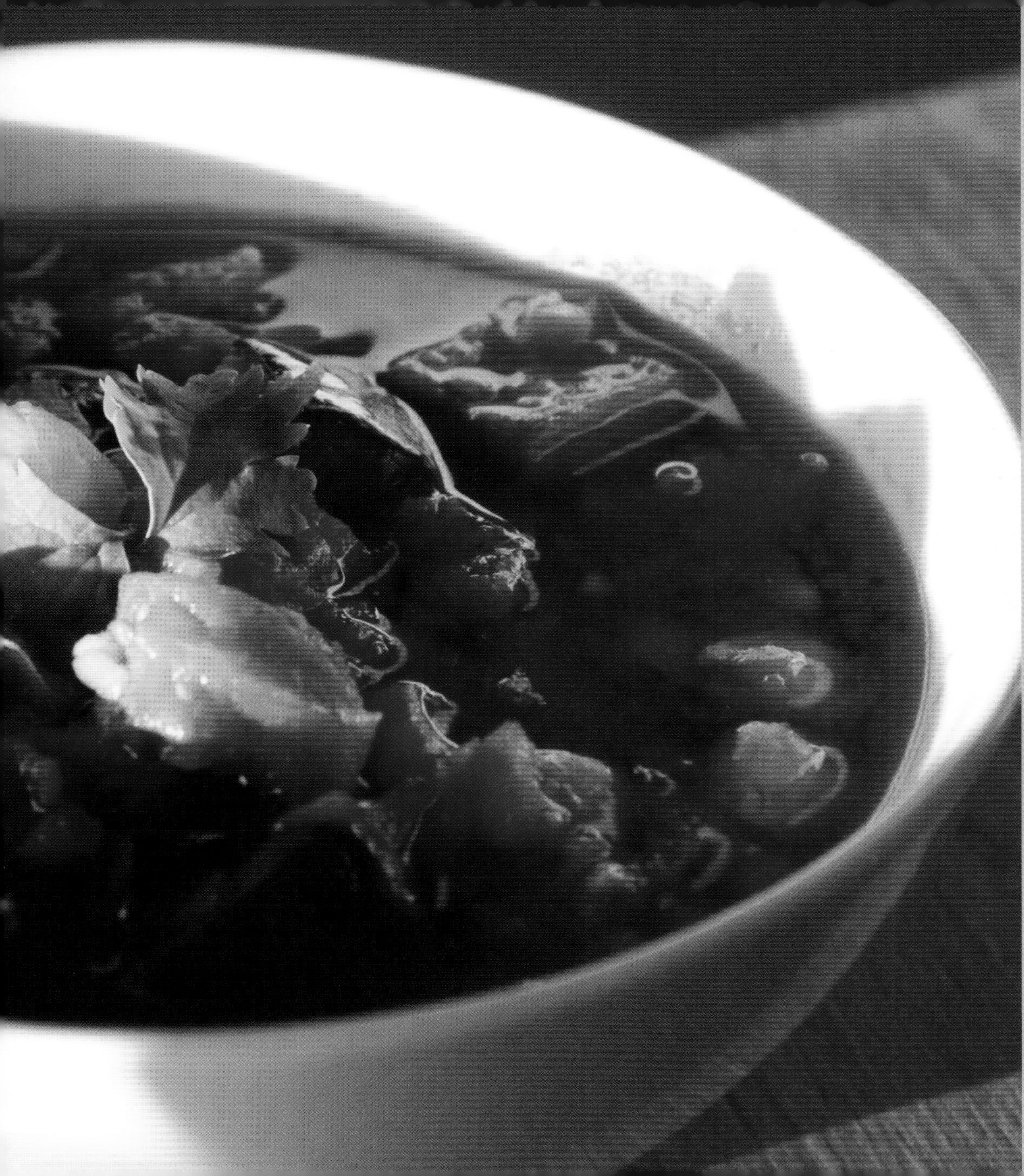

soup

Soup

There is nothing better on a blustery day than bundling up inside and eating a warm bowl of soup. And while it is said that soup season tends to be in the fall and winter, you can eat soup any time of year. The problem I used to face when making soup was that the recipes usually made enough to feed a small army. Over the years, I have learned two lessons in making soup for one: being financial savvy and removing the curse of the leftovers.

First, I have found that it is usually a bit of a drain on the pocketbook to buy ingredients for a soup. Soups tend to have a few more ingredients than other dishes, making them a bit more expensive, so any ease of the financial strain is always welcome. The beauty of these nine soup recipes is they are tailored to a single's budget, helping you to stretch the use of several ingredients.

Second, the problem in cooking soup for one usually lies in the leftovers. Having soup leftovers that provide at least three to five additional meals will lead you to get sick of the soup rather quickly. These recipes are specifically tailored to serve one, so your days of overexposure to one soup are over.

Ingredients

In general, soups tend to have similar ingredients. While you may notice that there are more ingredients for soups than for other dishes in this cookbook, you will also notice a lot of crossover among the different soups. While you only use one half of a carrot, onion, or stalk of celery in one recipe, you can actually use the rest of the carrot, onion, or stalk of celery to make another soup, thus giving you some variety. As a basis, here are some general items you will want to have on hand when you make a majority of the soups mentioned in this book:

- Stock—chicken broth, beef broth
- Vegetables—onions, tomatoes, celery stalk, carrots
- Garnish—fresh cilantro, parsley

Let's talk a little bit more about stock. Some people like to cook and store homemade stock. I have included a recipe below in case you want to make your own. This process takes about four to five hours to complete.

Chicken Stock

- leftover bones and skin of poultry or beef
- 1 large onion, chopped to fit in pan
- 3–5 carrots, chopped to fit in pan
- 3–5 celery stalks, chopped to fit in pan
- 3 Tbsp. minced garlic
- 1 Tbsp. black peppercorns (or pepper)
- 3 bay leaves
- 2 Tbsp. thyme

1. Put leftover bones and skin of poultry or beef into a large stock pot. (For a richer flavor, roast the skin, bones, and vegetables for about 45 minutes in the oven at 450 degrees before adding to the stock pot.)
2. Add onion, carrots, celery, garlic, and peppercorns. Cover with water. Bring to a boil. Reduce heat to a simmer and cook uncovered for 4 hours.
3. Strain stock through a small mesh colander to remove herbs and excess material.
4. Refrigerate for 2 hours and skim the excess fat accumulated on the surface.
5. Place the stock in containers and store in the refrigerator or freezer.

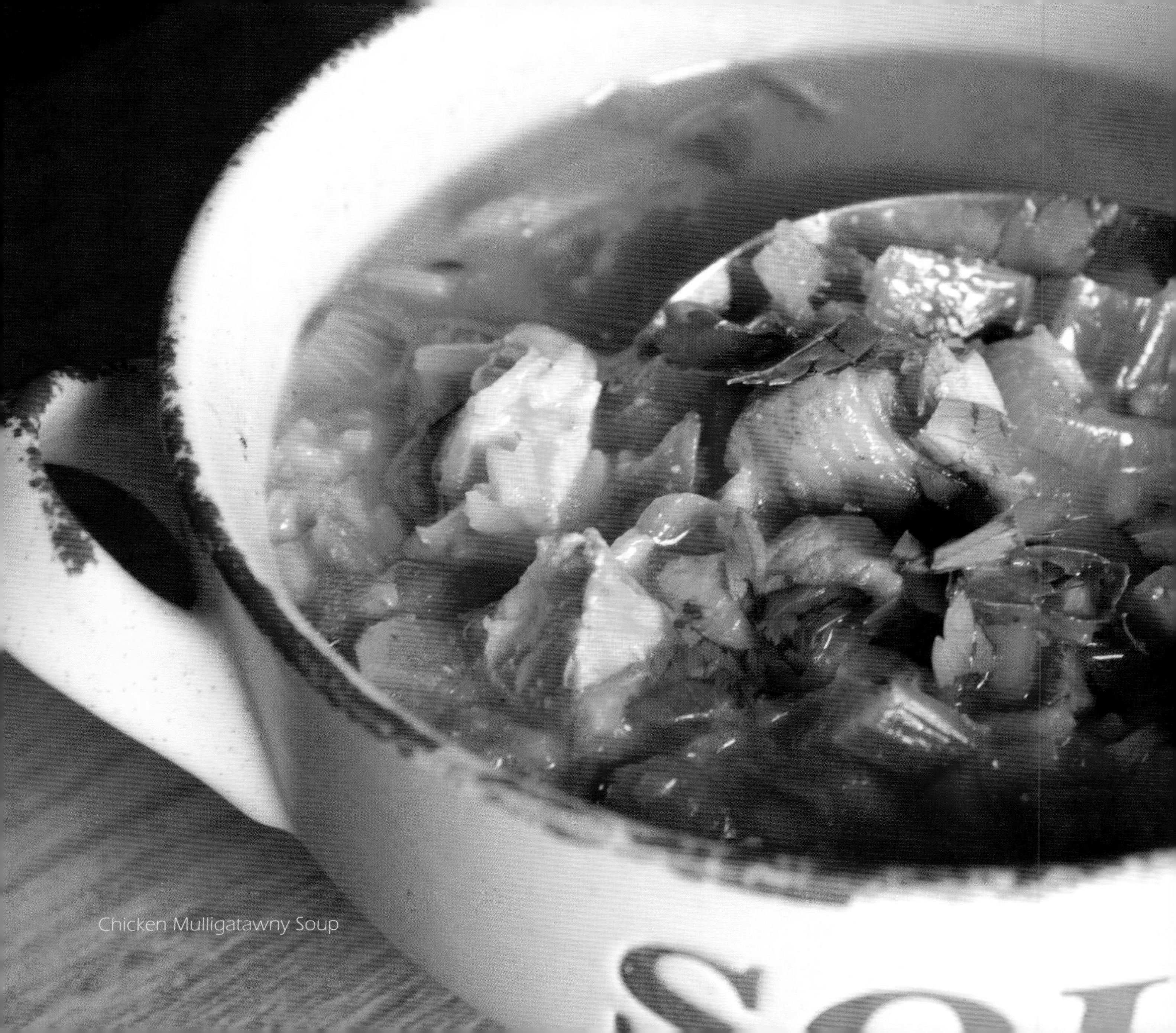

Chicken Mulligatawny Soup

Chicken Mulligatawny Soup

- 2 tsp. unsalted butter
- ½ cup **chicken breast**, cubed
- ¼ tsp. garlic, minced
- ¼ cup **yellow onion**, chopped
- ¼ cup **celery**, chopped
- ¼ cup **carrot**, chopped
- ¼ cup **granny smith apple**, chopped
- 1 ½ cup chicken broth
- 1 tsp. curry powder
- 1 Tbsp. lemon juice
- pinch of ground cloves
- pinch of salt and pepper
- 2 Tbsp. long grain white rice
- ¼ cup **plain yogurt**
- 2 tsp. **fresh cilantro**

1. Melt 1 tsp. butter in a medium skillet. Add chicken and garlic. Sauté for 5–7 minutes over medium-low heat until chicken is lightly browned. Set aside.
2. In the same skillet, add 1 tsp. butter, onion, celery, carrot, and apple. Sauté for 5–7 minutes over medium-low heat or until onion becomes translucent.
3. In a medium saucepan, add broth, curry, lemon juice, cloves, salt, pepper, chicken, and vegetables. Bring to a boil. Reduce to a simmer and add rice. Cook, uncovered, for 15–20 minutes.
4. Stir in yogurt and let simmer for another 5 minutes. Garnish with cilantro.

Lentil Soup

- 1 Tbsp. olive oil
- ¼ cup **carrot**, chopped
- ¼ cup **celery**, chopped
- ¼ cup **yellow onion**, chopped
- 1 tsp. garlic, minced
- pinch of salt and pepper
- ¼ tsp. dried thyme
- ½ cup **tomato**, chopped
- 1½ cup chicken broth
- ¼ cup fresh lentils
- 1½ tsp. white wine vinegar

1. In a medium saucepan, heat olive oil over medium heat. Add carrot, celery, onion, garlic, salt, and pepper. Sauté over medium-low heat for 5–7 minutes, until onion is translucent. Add thyme. Continue cooking for 3–5 minutes, until vegetables are soft.
2. Add tomatoes, chicken broth, and lentils. Bring to a boil. Reduce heat and simmer, partially covered, for 20 minutes. Stir in white wine vinegar.

Shrimp Gazpacho

- 2 Tbsp. olive oil
- 4–6 oz. **shrimp**, peeled and deveined (no tail)
- 1 cup **tomatoes**, chopped
- ¼ cup **red onion**, chopped
- 1 tsp. garlic, minced
- ¼ cup **cucumbers**, chopped
- ¼ cup **green bell pepper**, chopped
- ¼ cup **celery**, chopped
- ½ cup tomato juice
- 1½ tsp. **tomato paste**
- dash of salt and pepper
- 1½ tsp. red wine vinegar
- ¼ cup **avocado**, chopped
- 1 Tbsp. **fresh cilantro**, chopped

1. Heat 1 Tbsp. olive oil in a small skillet. Add shrimp and season with salt and pepper. Sauté over medium-low heat for 3–5 minutes, until shrimp are browned on both sides and opaque in the center.
2. In a food processor or blender, mix 1 Tbsp. olive oil, tomatoes, onion, garlic, cucumbers, bell pepper, and celery. Add tomato juice, tomato paste, vinegar, salt, and pepper. Process until soupy.
3. Pour mixture into a bowl. Add shrimp and garnish with avocado and cilantro.

Chicken Posole Soup

- 2 cups water
- ½ cup **chicken breast**
- 1 Tbsp. olive oil
- ¼ cup **yellow onion**, chopped
- 1 tsp. garlic, minced
- ½ cup **stewed tomatoes**, canned
- ¼ tsp. chili powder
- ½ tsp. dried oregano
- 1 cup chicken broth
- ½ cup white hominy, canned
- pinch of salt and pepper
- 1 **radish**, thinly sliced
- 1 tsp. **fresh parsley**

1. Bring 2 cups water to a boil in a medium saucepan. Add chicken. Cover and simmer for 10–12 minutes, until cooked through. Transfer chicken to a platter and let cool. Shred chicken with a fork.
2. Meanwhile, heat olive oil in another medium saucepan and add onions. Sauté for 5–7 minutes over medium-low heat, stirring occasionally, until onions are translucent.
3. Add garlic, stewed tomatoes, chili powder, and oregano. Add chicken broth, ½ cup water, and hominy. Bring to a boil and then reduce heat to a simmer and cook, uncovered, for 15–20 minutes.
4. Add shredded chicken and season with salt and pepper to taste. Garnish with radish slices and parsley.

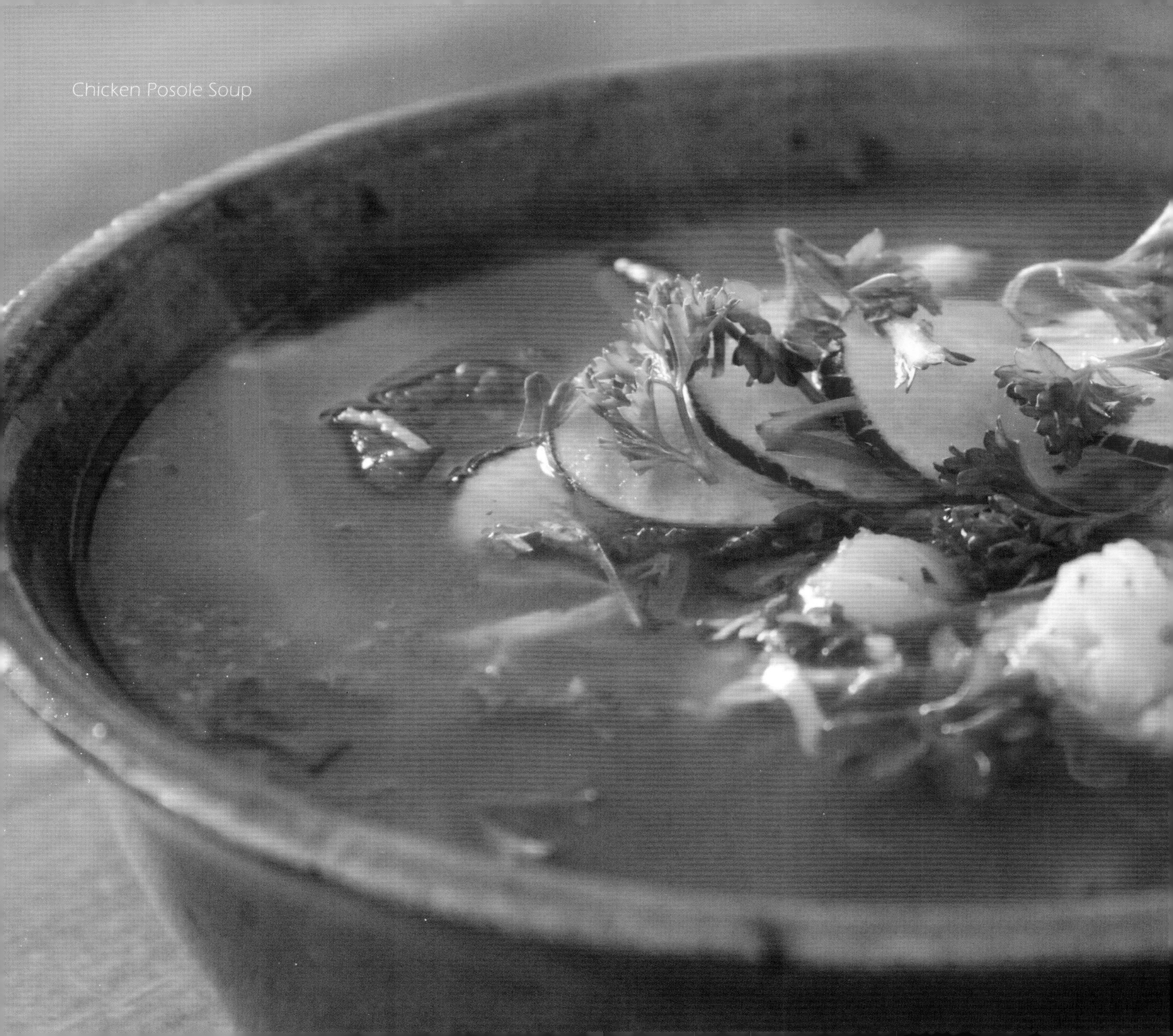
Chicken Posole Soup

French Onion Soup

- ¼ **French baguette**, ½ inch slices
- ½ **yellow onion**, thinly sliced
- 1 Tbsp. unsalted butter
- ½ tsp. sugar
- ½ tsp. flour
- ¼ cup water
- 1 Tbsp. white wine (optional)
- 1 cup chicken broth
- ¼ cup **apple cider**
- ¼ tsp. thyme
- 1 slice **Swiss cheese**

1. Preheat oven to 325 degrees. Cut two ½-inch thick slices from baguette and lay on baking sheet. Toast in oven for about 10 minutes. Reserve the rest of the baguette to serve with the soup as a side.
2. Slice onion into thin round circles. The middle slices of an onion are the best.
3. Melt butter in a medium saucepan over medium-low heat. Add sugar and onions. Stir occasionally so onions do not burn. Sauté for 5–10 minutes over medium-low heat or until onions are golden brown.
4. Stir in flour, water, white wine, chicken broth, and apple cider. Bring to a boil. Reduce heat to simmer. Add thyme. Cover soup and let cook for 10 minutes.
5. Top toasted baguette with Swiss cheese and return baking pan to oven for another 2–4 minutes, until cheese is melted.
6. Ladle soup into bowl and place toasted bread on top of the soup.

Split Pea Soup

- ½ Tbsp. unsalted butter
- ¼ cup **yellow onion**, chopped
- ¼ cup **carrot**, chopped
- ¼ cup **celery**, chopped
- ½ tsp. dried oregano
- dash of salt and pepper
- 1 cup chicken broth
- ½ cup green split peas
- 1 ham bone (and extra ham from bone)
- 1 cup water
- 1½ tsp. lemon juice

1. In a medium saucepan, heat butter over medium heat and add onions. Stir occasionally. Sauté over medium-low heat for 3–5 minutes. Add carrots, celery, oregano, and dash of salt and pepper. Cook for 5–7 minutes, until vegetables are soft.
2. Add broth, split peas, ham bone, and 1 cup water. Bring to a boil. Reduce heat to a simmer and cook covered about 40 minutes, until peas are soft.
3. Remove ham bone from soup. Puree soup in a blender and return to pot. Add bits of ham from ham bone and simmer for 5 minutes. Add lemon juice and salt and pepper to taste.

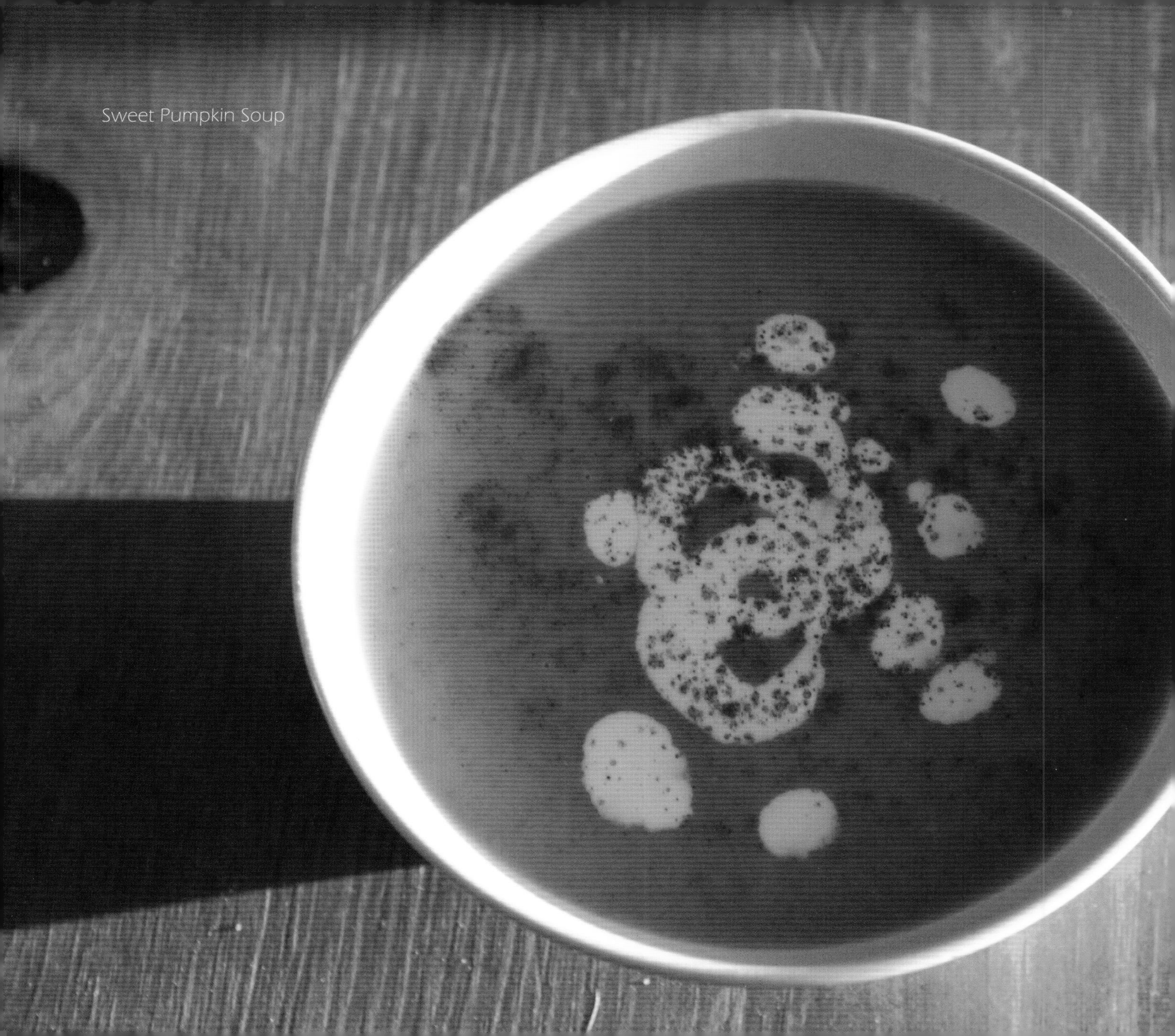

Sweet Pumpkin Soup

Sweet Pumpkin Soup

- ½ cup **apple cider**
- ½ cup water
- 2 Tbsp. sugar
- ¾ cup pumpkin puree
- ½ tsp. pumpkin pie spice
- ¼ cup **heavy whipping cream**
- ¼ tsp. cinnamon

1. In a medium saucepan, combine apple cider, ½ cup water, sugar, pumpkin puree, and pumpkin pie spice. Bring to a boil. Reduce heat to low and simmer uncovered for 5 minutes.
2. Stir in heavy cream and cinnamon. Simmer for 3–5 more minutes. Transfer soup to a bowl. Garnish with cinnamon and a few drops of whipping cream.

Thai-Chicken Coconut Soup

- 1 Tbsp. olive oil
- ½ cup **chicken breast**, cubed
- ½ tsp. garlic, minced
- ¼ medium **orange** (and **orange zest**)
- 1 cup **coconut milk**
- ½ cup chicken broth
- 1 tsp. Asian fish sauce
- 1 pinch of ground ginger
- 2 oz. **button mushrooms**
- salt and pepper to taste
- 3 tsp. **fresh cilantro**

1. In a medium skillet, add olive oil, chicken, and garlic. Sauté over medium-low heat for 5–7 minutes, until lightly brown. Set chicken aside.
2. In a medium saucepan, combine orange (and zest), coconut milk, broth, fish sauce, and ginger. Bring to a boil. Add mushrooms. Cook uncovered for 5 minutes.
3. Season to taste with salt and pepper. Garnish with cilantro.

Tomato and Eggplant Soup

- ¼ cup **tomato**, chopped
- ¼ cup **eggplant**, cubed (without skin)
- ¼ cup **yellow onion**, chopped
- 1 tsp. garlic, minced
- 1 Tbsp. olive oil
- ½ tsp. thyme
- ½ cup water
- 1½ cup chicken broth
- ¼ cup **chickpeas**, drained
- salt and pepper to taste
- 1 tsp. **fresh cilantro**

1. Preheat oven to 400 degrees. Place tomato on one side of a baking sheet. On the other side of the baking sheet, add eggplant, onion, and garlic. Drizzle with olive oil. Bake for 45 minutes.
2. In a small saucepan, add roasted tomatoes, thyme, water, and chicken broth. Bring to a boil. Reduce heat and simmer for 10 minutes.
3. Working in batches, puree soup in blender until smooth. Return puree to saucepan. Add roasted eggplant/onion mixture, chickpeas, salt, and pepper. Garnish with cilantro.

Tortilla Soup

Base

- ½ tsp. unsalted butter
- 2 Tbsp. **yellow onion**, chopped
- ¼ tsp. garlic, minced
- 2 Tbsp. **carrot**, chopped
- 2 Tbsp. **celery**, chopped
- dash of salt and pepper
- 1 cup chicken broth
- 1 Tbsp. **lime juice**
- 1 cup water
- ¼ cup **chicken breast**, cubed

Add-ins

- ¼ cup **avocado**, chopped
- ¼ cup **tomato**, chopped
- 1 Tbsp. **sour cream**
- ¼ cup **cheddar cheese**, shredded
- 1 Tbsp. **fresh cilantro**
- tortilla chips, crushed or whole

1. In a medium saucepan, heat butter over medium heat and add onions and garlic. Sauté over medium-low heat for 3–5 minutes, stirring occasionally.
2. Add carrots, celery, oregano, and a dash of salt and pepper. Sauté over medium-low heat for 5–7 minutes, until vegetables are soft.
3. Add chicken broth, lime juice, and water. Bring to a boil. Maintain at a boil for 15–20 minutes.
4. Place add-ins, except tortilla chips, in a bowl. Cover with soup. Place tortilla chips on top.

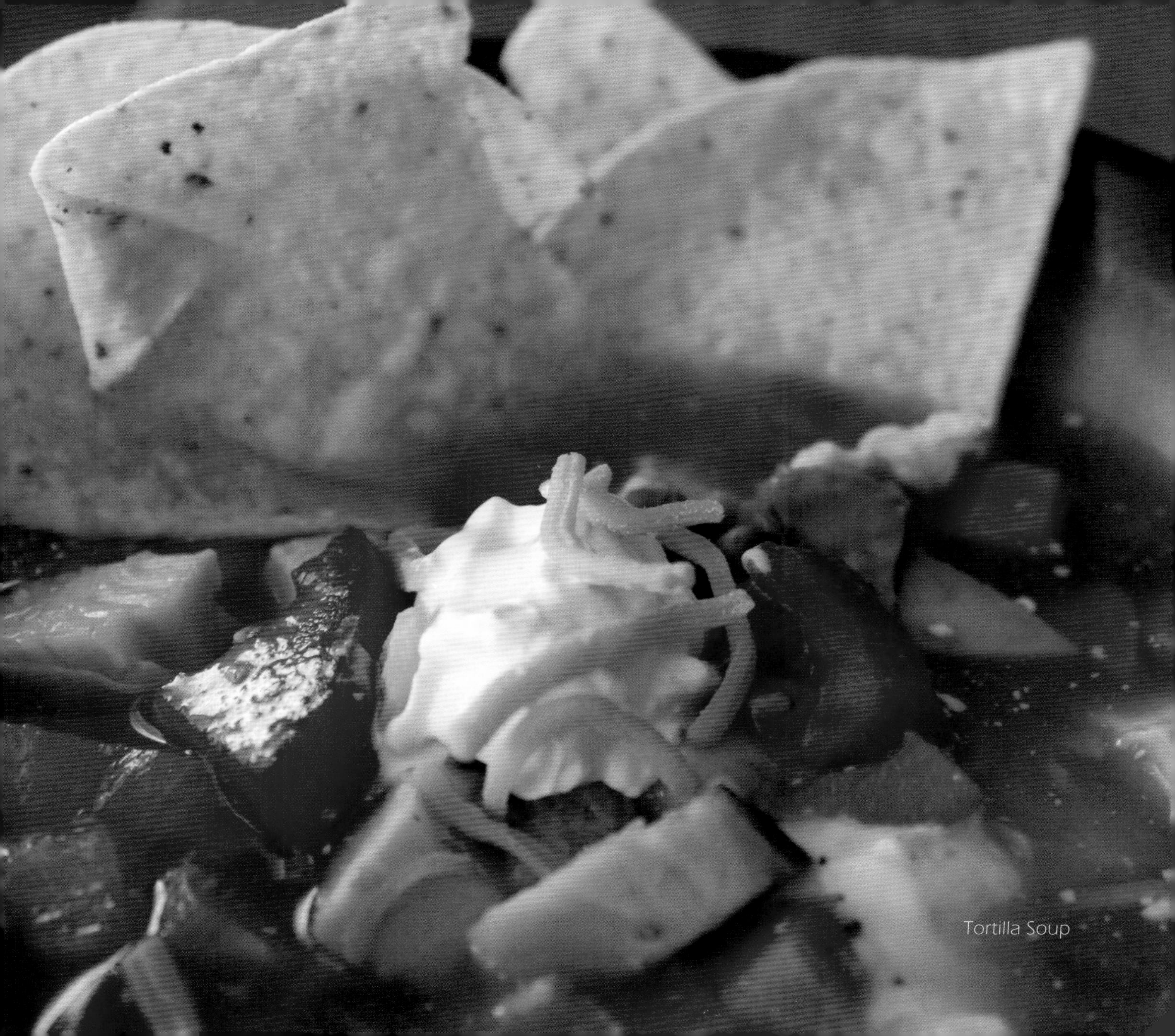

Tortilla Soup

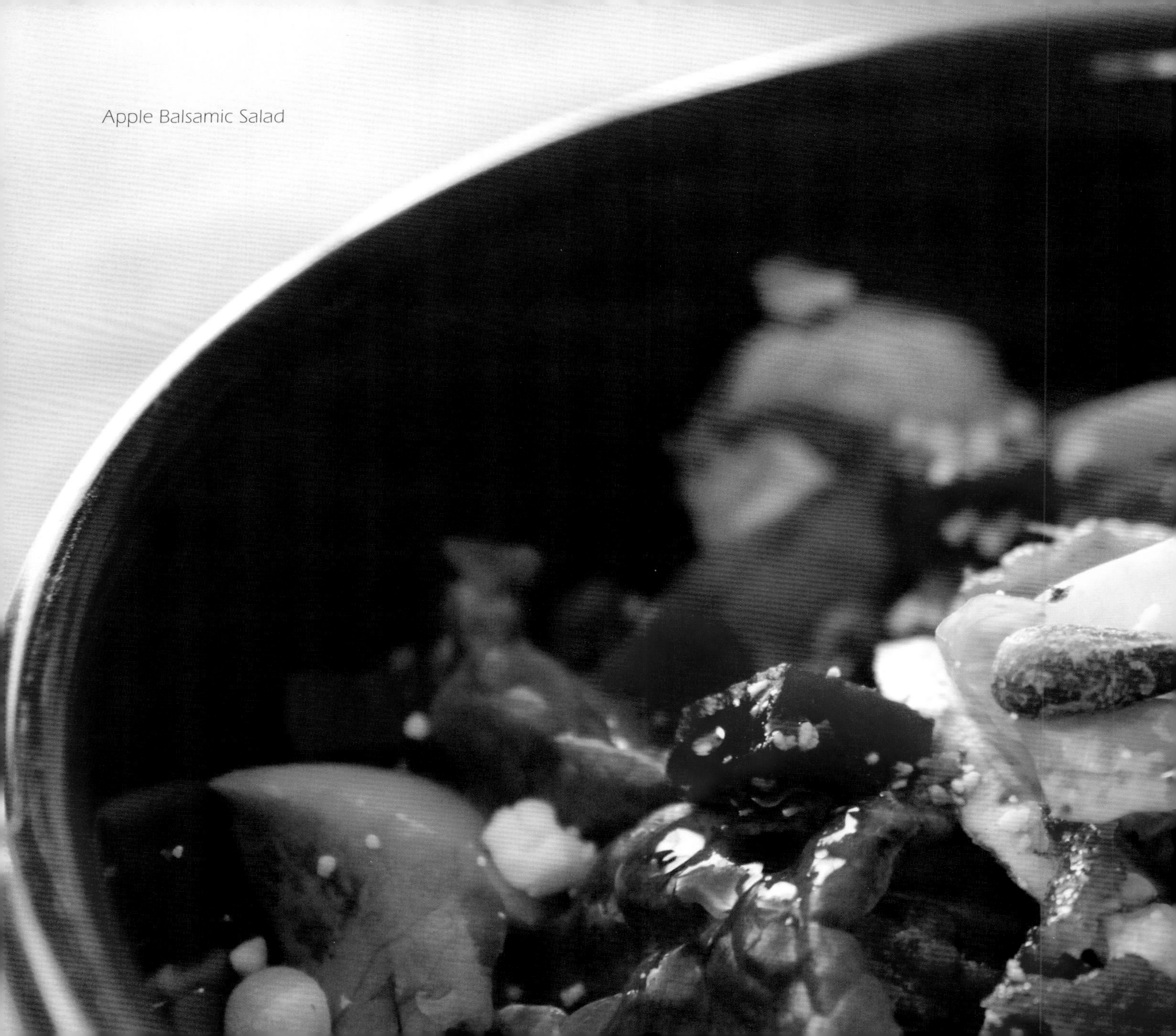

Apple Balsamic Salad

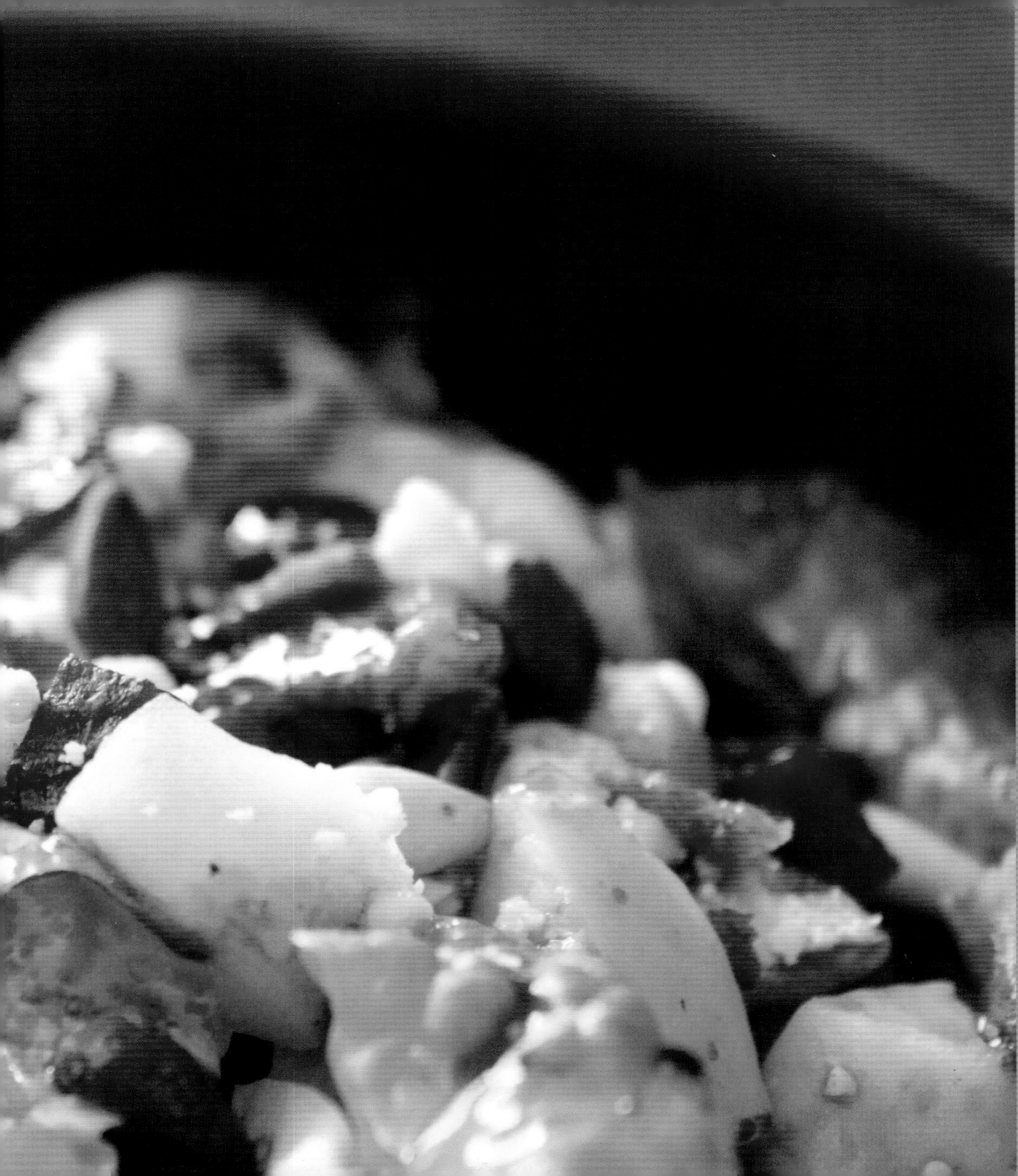

Salad

Salad

Salads are a single chef's best friend. They allow you to bring in the hodgepodge of excess ingredients that you have used for other recipes and put them to good, healthy use. However, I need to point out that its semblance to a hodgepodge is what makes a salad actually taste good. I've seen my fair share of attempts to throw a salad together go very, very wrong. Who knew that tomato paste and cantaloupe wouldn't work together in a salad? After many failed and successful experiments, I developed this section on salads to help you use excess ingredients with confidence. But before we dive right into the recipes, we should review some lettuce basics.

Lettuce Basics

There are many types of lettuce. I have tried to keep this cookbook to a select few so that you don't have too much excess. But let's review the basic types of lettuce, in case you would like to switch out a lettuce type that I have suggested for another.

1. **Arugula**—This leaf has a peppery, pungent flavor and a unique shape. The flavor intensity varies with the size of the leaf. The bigger the leaf, the stronger the flavor. Arugula is often mixed with other milder greens to provide for a richer taste and greater aesthetic appeal. The downfall is that this type of lettuce is not typically found in the common grocery store, but when you can find it, I highly recommend using it with salads that have a sweet aftertaste to balance the flavor.
2. **Chard**—This leaf usually has large leaves with a red rib down the center and a spinachlike flavor. You can typically find it in the average grocery store.

3. **Endive**—This type of lettuce has a mildly bitter flavor, and its unique leaf shape can add visual stimuli to a salad, even if all you do is mix it in with other leaves. You might see it called "curly endive" in the store.

4. **Iceberg**—This type of leaf is also known as a crisphead because it is tight and dense, resembling cabbage. Typically, iceberg lettuce is not as nutritionally rich as other options, but it is a common choice and can always be found in the grocery store.

5. **Radicchio**—This type of lettuce is bitter and has a peppery taste when eaten alone. It has red leaves and adds visually to a salad, but is usually a mix-in with other types of lettuce because of its steep cost.

6. **Romaine**—This lettuce has large and crisp leaves, a firm rib down the center, and a slightly sharp flavor. There are two types of Romaine leaves: green and red leaf. This cookbook mainly calls for Romaine lettuce, because it has a far-reaching use for other recipes as well as salads, and is commonly found in stores. Hopefully, this will allow you to stretch your dollar.

7. **Spinach**—This leaf is more rounded and has a mildly hearty flavor. This leaf is highly nutritious, being extremely rich in antioxidants and iron.

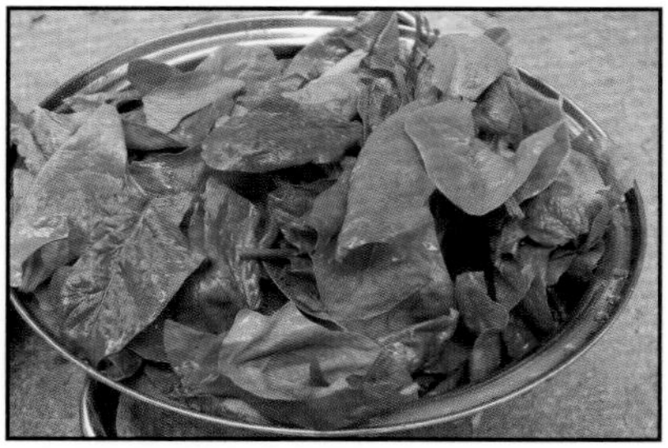

Spinach

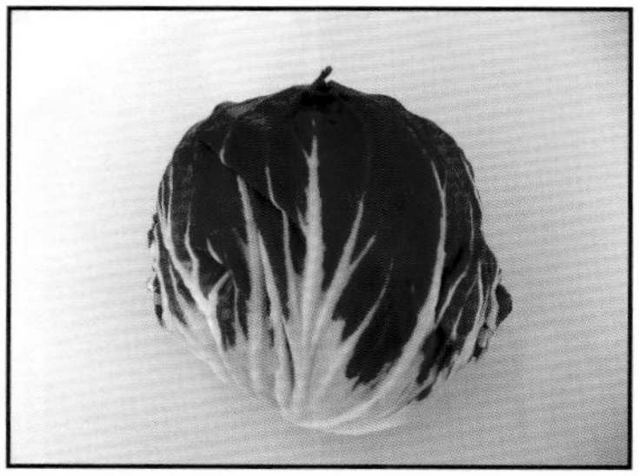

Radicchio

Orange Ginger Salad

Salad

- 2 Tbsp. **stir fry beef**
- 2 handfuls **red leaf Romaine lettuce**
- 2 Tbsp. **dried cranberries**
- ¼ cup **mushrooms**, sliced
- ¼ cup **orange**, peeled and sliced
- 2 Tbsp. **green onion**, sliced
- 1 tsp. **sesame seeds**

Dressing

- ¼ tsp. garlic, minced
- ½ tsp. **fresh ginger root**, minced
- 2 tsp. extra virgin olive oil
- 1 tsp. rice vinegar
- 1 tsp. soy sauce
- 1 tsp. honey

1. Heat oil in a small skillet over medium-high heat. Add beef and cook for 2–4 minutes, stirring frequently, until beef is cooked through. Remove beef from skillet and let cool.
2. Toss together contents of salad in a medium bowl or on a plate.
3. Mix together dressing ingredients in a small cup. Stir well and toss with salad. Use extra orange slices for garnish.

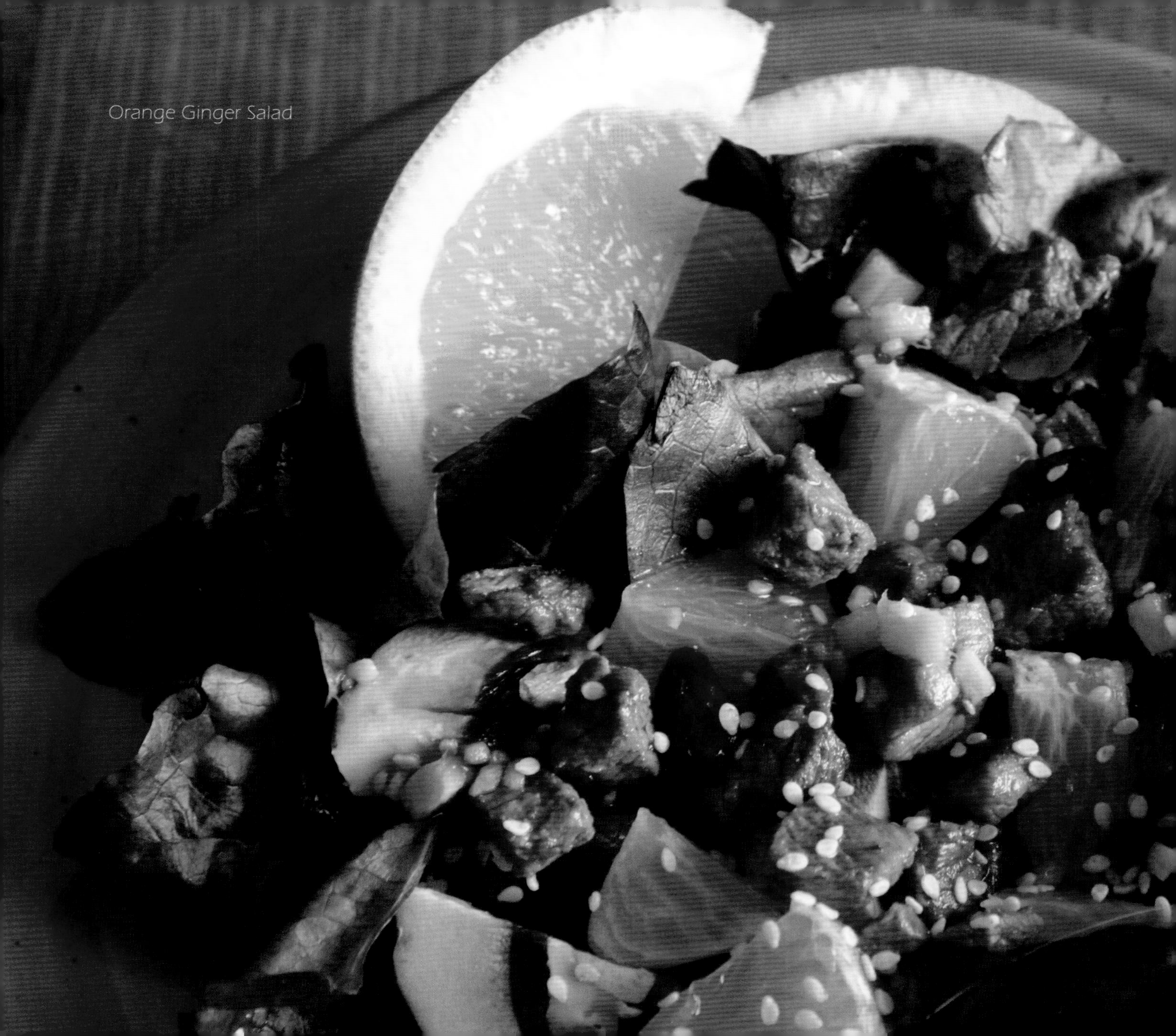
Orange Ginger Salad

Blueberry Pear Salad

Salad

- 2 handfuls **red leaf Romaine lettuce**
- ¼ cup cooked **turkey**, chopped or shredded
- ¼ cup **blueberries**
- ¼ cup pear, chopped
- 1 Tbsp. **fresh mozzarella cheese**, shredded
- 1 Tbsp. **sunflower seeds**
- 1 Tbsp. **bean sprouts**

Dressing

- 1 Tbsp. **plain yogurt**
- 1 tsp. **raspberry vinegar**
- ½ tsp. tarragon
- 1½ tsp. brown sugar

1. Toss together contents of salad in a medium bowl or on a plate.
2. Mix together contents of dressing in a small cup. Stir well and toss with salad.

Caesar Salad

Salad

- ½ **chicken breast**
- salt and pepper
- 1 Tbsp. olive oil
- 2 handfuls **green leaf Romaine lettuce**
- ¼ cup croutons
- 2 Tbsp. **Parmesan cheese**, grated

Dressing

- ¼ cup **mayonnaise**
- 1 tsp. lemon juice
- ¼ tsp. **Worcestershire sauce**
- ¼ tsp. garlic, minced
- 1 tsp. milk
- dash of salt and pepper

1. Heat grill to medium-high. Season chicken with salt and pepper. Grill chicken breast for about 5 minutes on each side, until golden brown on both sides and no longer pink in the center. Remove chicken from heat and let cool. Cut chicken julienne.
2. Toss together contents of salad in a medium bowl or on a plate.
3. Mix together contents of dressing in a small cup. Stir well and toss with salad.

Citrus Salad

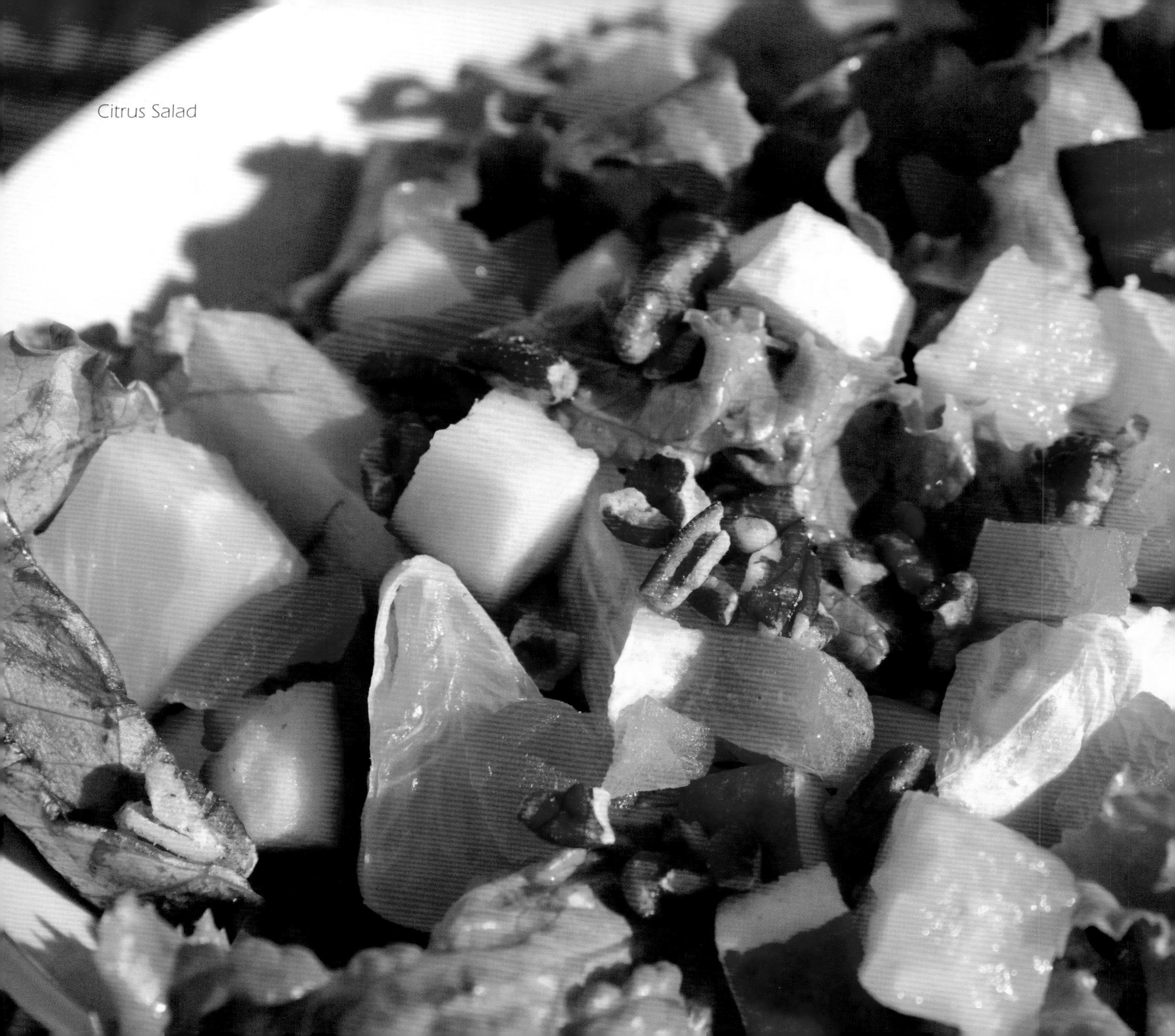

Citrus Salad

Salad

- 2 handfuls **green leaf Romaine lettuce**
- ¼ cup **orange**, peeled and chopped
- ¼ cup gala or red delicious **apple**, chopped
- 2 Tbsp. **dried apricots**, chopped
- 2 Tbsp. **pineapple**, peeled and chopped
- 1 Tbsp. **walnuts**, chopped

Vinaigrette

- 1 Tbsp. extra virgin olive oil
- 1 tsp. **orange juice**
- 1 tsp. lemon juice
- 1 tsp. honey
- 1 tsp. **fresh basil**, chopped
- 2 tsp. white wine vinegar
- dash of salt and pepper

1. Toss together contents of salad in a medium bowl or on a plate.
2. Mix together contents of vinaigrette in a small cup. Stir well and toss with salad.

Honey Bacon Salad

Salad

- 1 strip **bacon**
- 2 handfuls **red leaf Romaine lettuce**
- 2 Tbsp. canned **beets**, chopped
- 1 hard-boiled egg, chopped
- ¼ cup **mushrooms**, sliced
- 1 Tbsp. **almonds**, slivered
- 1 tsp. **Parmesan cheese**, grated

Dressing

- 1 Tbsp. extra virgin olive oil
- 1 Tbsp. balsamic vinegar
- ¼ tsp. tarragon
- ½ tsp. lemon juice
- dash of salt and pepper

1. Cook bacon in a small skillet until lightly browned, about 2 minutes on each side. Remove from skillet and let cool. Pat down bacon with a paper towel to remove excess grease. Crumble.
2. Toss together contents of salad in a medium bowl or on a plate.
3. Mix together contents of dressing in a small cup. Stir well and toss with salad.

Apple Balsamic Salad

Salad

- 1 ½ Tbsp. toasted **pine nuts**
- 1 strip **bacon**
- 2 handfuls **red leaf Romaine lettuce**
- ¼ cup **mushrooms**, chopped
- ¼ cup **granny smith apple**, chopped
- 2 Tbsp. **grapes**, chopped
- 2 Tbsp. canned **beets**, chopped
- 2 Tbsp. **feta cheese**

Vinaigrette

- 1 Tbsp. extra virgin olive oil
- 1 tsp. maple syrup or brown sugar
- 2 tsp. balsamic vinegar
- dash of salt and pepper

1. Place pine nuts on small baking pan and broil for 1–2 minutes on each side, until toasted.
2. Cook bacon in a small skillet, until lightly browned, about 2 minutes on each side. Remove from skillet and let cool. Pat down bacon with a paper towel to remove excess grease. Crumble.
3. Toss together contents of salad in a medium bowl or on a plate.
4. Mix contents of vinaigrette in a small cup. Stir well and toss with salad.

Lemon Dill Salad

Salad

- ¼ cup **salmon**
- 2 handfuls **green leaf Romaine lettuce**
- 2 Tbsp. **zucchini**, chopped
- 2 Tbsp. **carrots**, chopped
- ¼ cup **red onions**, chopped
- 1–2 Tbsp. **kalamata olives**
- 1 Tbsp. **almonds**, slivered

Dressing

- 1 Tbsp. **plain yogurt**
- 1 tsp. lemon juice
- ¼ tsp. dill weed
- ½ tsp. sugar
- 1 tsp. white wine vinegar

1. In a small skillet, cook salmon for 3–4 minutes on each side. Remove from skillet and cool. Break into pieces.
2. Toss together contents of salad in a medium bowl or on a plate.
3. Mix together contents of dressing in a small cup. Stir well and toss with salad.

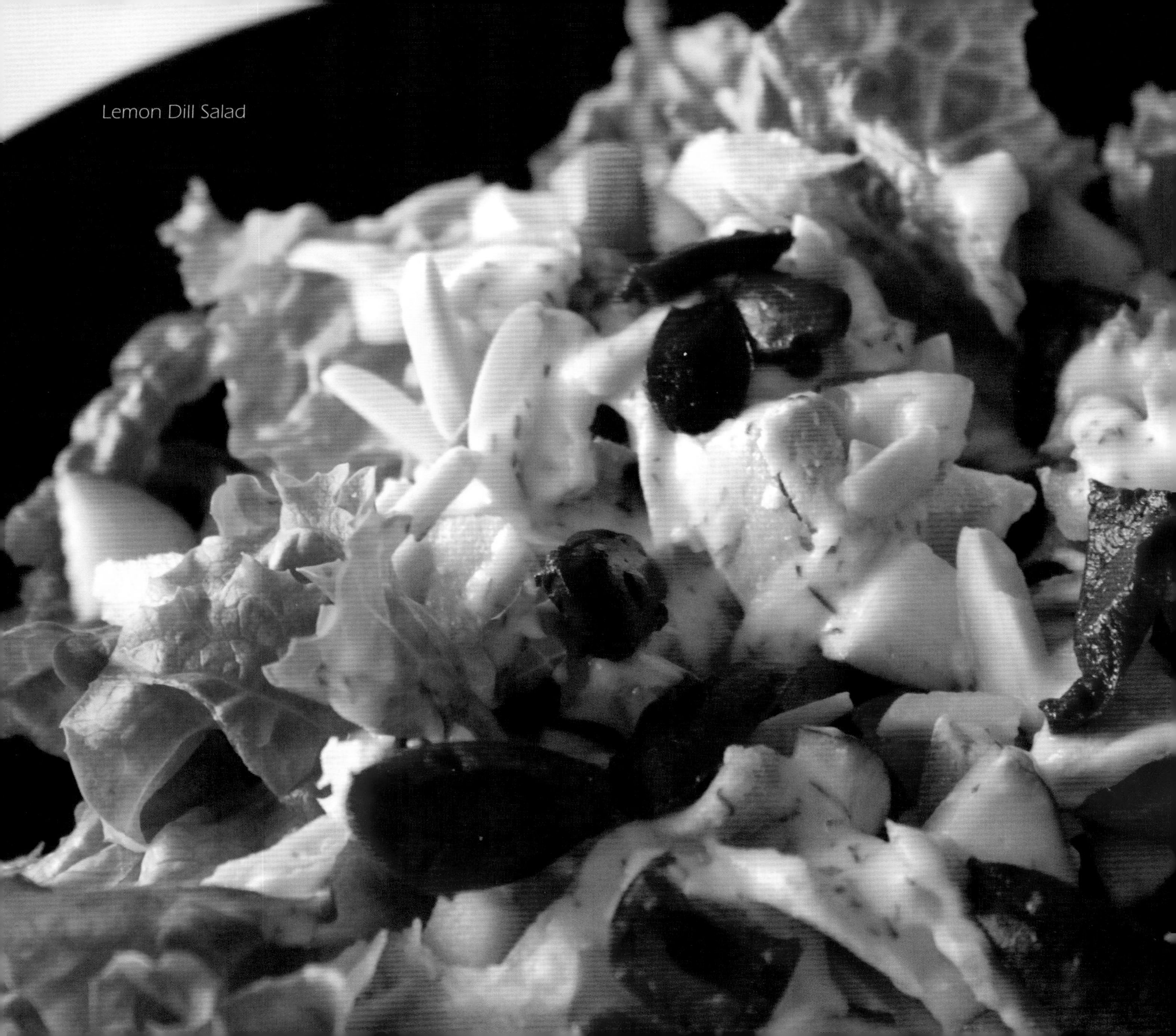

Lemon Dill Salad

Raspberry Sunflower Salad

Salad

- 2 handfuls **green leaf Romaine lettuce**
- ¼ cup **turkey**, shredded
- ¼ cup **red onion**, sliced into rings
- 2 Tbsp. **mushrooms**, sliced
- 1 Tbsp. **raspberries**, sliced
- 2 Tbsp. **dried cranberries**
- 2 Tbsp. Spanish olives, sliced
- 1 Tbsp. **fresh mozzarella cheese**, shredded
- 1 Tbsp. **sunflower seeds**

Vinaigrette

- 1 Tbsp. **raspberry preserves**
- 1 tsp. **raspberry vinegar**
- ½ tsp. lemon juice
- 1 tsp. olive oil
- 1 tsp. **fresh mint**, chopped

1. Toss together contents of salad in a medium bowl or on a plate.
2. Mix together contents of vinaigrette in a small cup. Stir well and toss with salad.

Taco Salad

- 1 tsp. olive oil
- 2 handfuls **iceberg lettuce**
- ½ **chicken breast**, shredded
- ¼ cup **black beans**
- ¼ cup **avocado**, chopped
- ¼ cup **tomato**, chopped
- 2 Tbsp. **black olives**, chopped
- 1 **radish**, chopped
- 2 Tbsp. **chickpeas**, chopped
- 2 Tbsp. **cheddar cheese**, shredded
- 2 Tbsp. **sour cream**
- ¼ cup salsa

1. Add oil and chicken to medium skillet. Sauté chicken over medium-low heat, 5–7 minutes on each side, until cooked through. Set aside to cool. Shred chicken by pulling apart with fingers or a fork.
2. Toss together contents of salad in a medium bowl or on a plate. For best results, layer the salad in the order the ingredients are given.

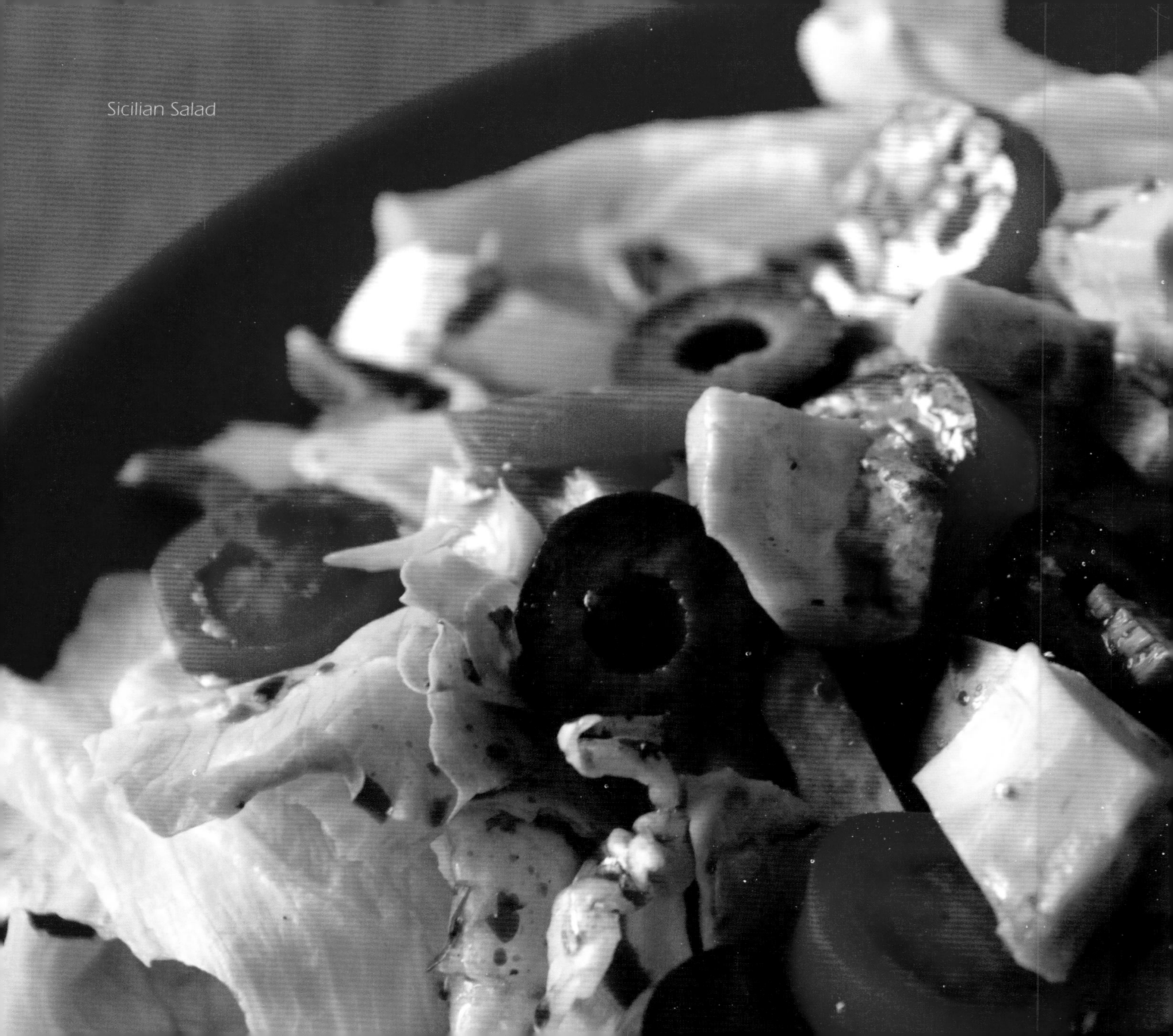
Sicilian Salad

Sicilian Salad

Salad

- 2 handfuls **iceberg lettuce**
- 1 **radish**, thinly sliced
- ¼ cup **cucumber**, chopped
- ¼ cup **mushrooms**, sliced
- 2 Tbsp. **black olives**, sliced
- ¼ cup **grape tomatoes**, sliced
- ¼ cup **avocado**, chopped

Vinaigrette

- 1 Tbsp. extra virgin olive oil
- 1 Tbsp. balsamic vinegar
- ¼ tsp. tarragon
- ½ tsp. lemon juice
- dash of salt and pepper

1. Toss together contents of salad in a medium bowl or on a plate.
2. Mix together contents of vinaigrette in a small cup. Stir well and toss with salad.

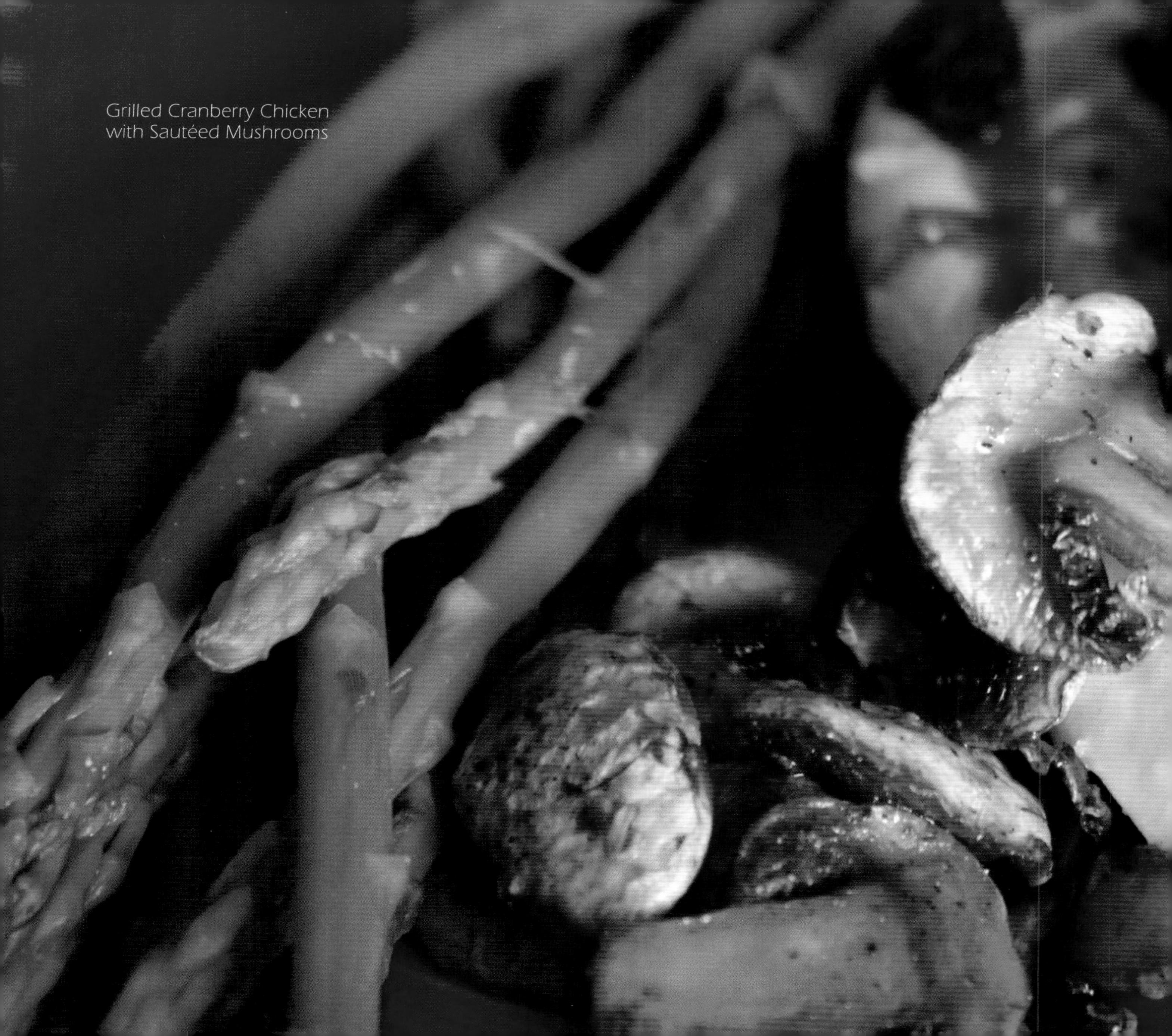

Grilled Cranberry Chicken
with Sautéed Mushrooms

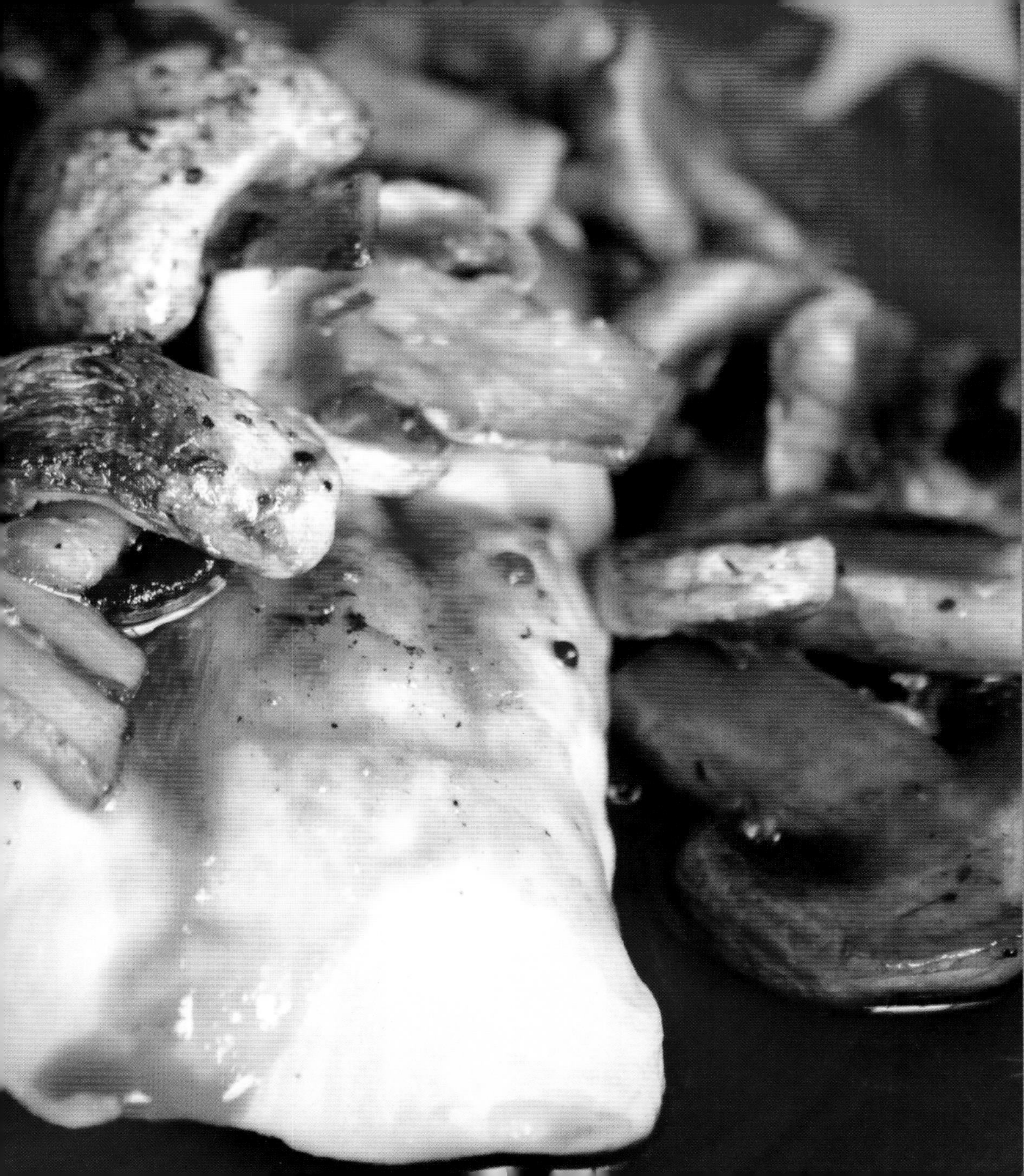

Poultry

Poultry

Poultry is often the default meat of the single lifestyle. When I first started cooking for myself, I would buy chicken without knowing what to do with it. Over the years, I have found some great ideas for glazes, rubs, and marinades that help flavor chicken.

Because poultry includes more than just chicken, I have included general cooking information on both chicken and turkey, even though this cookbook heavily favors chicken due to its common usage.

Chicken

There are many different ways to cook chicken, but I have found that three basic ways work best for the single lifestyle. Once you get good at cooking chicken, you can add most any glaze, marinade, or rub to make a great meal. Let's review the basic cooking methods for chicken:

1. **Sauté**—Season chicken with salt and pepper. In a small nonstick skillet, heat olive oil over medium-high heat. Add chicken and cook for 5–10 minutes on each side, until golden on the outside and opaque throughout (may differ with each recipe and the thickness of chicken).
2. **Grill**—Heat grill to medium-high. Season chicken breast with salt and pepper. Grill chicken, turning once, for about 5 minutes on each side (may differ with size of chicken breast), until golden brown on both sides and no longer pink in the center.
3. **Bake**—Preheat oven to 475 degrees. Line a rimmed baking sheet with foil. Place chicken

on prepared pan. Roast for 20–25 minutes, until chicken is deep brown on the outside and opaque throughout (may differ with each recipe).

Turkey

Cooking turkey is a challenge. Typically we eat turkey on special occasions, such as Thanksgiving, because we are not usually given cuts in the meat department that allow us to have portions of the bird, as we are with chicken. Regrettably, I was not able to figure a way of having something as delectable as a Thanksgiving turkey meal for one, but I have found some tips to help you incorporate turkey into your diet.

1. **Ground Turkey**—You may have seen ground turkey in the store. People argue that ground turkey is the healthy alternative to ground beef. However, in doing some research, I was able to find that lean ground beef and ground turkey are nearly identical nutrition-wise. However, turkey does tend to be a bit more bland and does require additional seasoning.
2. **Deli Sliced Turkey**—The reason so many people love sandwiches is because of turkey. A turkey sandwich is an American favorite. But buying sliced turkey is a bit harder. When you buy prepackaged sliced turkey, you may have initiated a race against the clock. For this reason, I go to the deli counter to get my meat sliced by the butcher. When you approach the butcher, have an idea of how many slices of turkey you will need for the upcoming week or two. I typically order two or three slices for one sandwich. By ordering the right amount, you spend less, waste less, and have better tasting turkey. It's the only way to go.

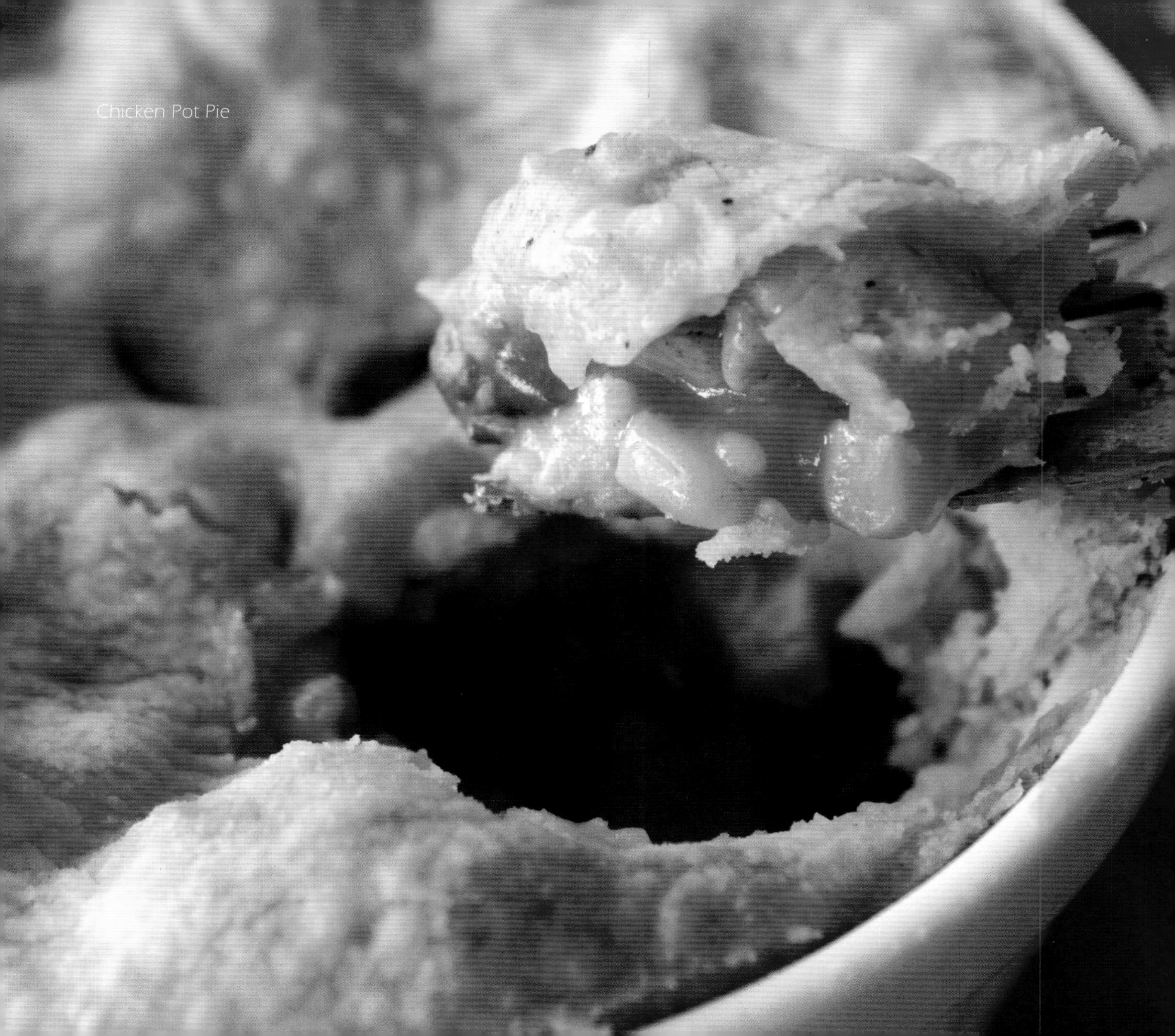
Chicken Pot Pie

Chicken Pot Pie

Pastry dough

- ¾ cup flour
- ¼ tsp. salt
- 1 ½ tsp. sugar
- 6 Tbsp. unsalted butter, room temp.
- ½ tsp. water

Chicken Mixture

- 1 Tbsp. unsalted butter
- ½ cup **chicken breast**, cubed
- ¼ cup **yellow onion**, diced
- 2 Tbsp. flour
- ¼ cup string beans
- ¼ cup **corn**
- ¼ tsp. thyme
- 1 cup chicken broth
- dash of salt and pepper
- 1 Tbsp. water
- 1 egg yolk

1. Preheat oven to 375 degrees. In a bowl combine flour, salt, and sugar. Add butter and water and mix until dough is ready to knead. Chill dough in the refrigerator for 30 minutes to set.
2. Meanwhile, in a medium skillet, melt butter over medium heat. Add chicken and onions and sauté for 5–7 minutes, until onions are soft. Add flour and salt to chicken mixture. Stir for about 2 minutes, until it becomes lightly golden.
3. Add chicken broth. Whisk constantly for 3–4 minutes, until mixture thickens. Reduce heat to low. Simmer mixture for 5 minutes. Mix in string beans, corn, and thyme. Season with salt and pepper.
4. Remove dough from refrigerator. Roll out dough on floured surface until ¼-inch thin. Use ¾ of the dough to place in bottom of a 5-inch ramekin.
5. Pour chicken mixture into a ramekin lined with dough. Cover mixture with remaining dough and cut vents in the dough cover.
6. In a small bowl, combine egg and 1 Tbsp. water. Brush top of dough with egg yolk mixture. Place ramekin on a baking sheet. Bake 35 minutes. Let cool for about 5 minutes.

BBQ Chicken

- dash of salt and ground pepper
- 2 Tbsp. **Worcestershire sauce**
- 2 Tbsp. red wine vinegar
- 2 Tbsp. olive oil
- 1 Tbsp. honey
- 1 tsp. **stone-ground mustard**
- ½ tsp. garlic minced
- 1 Tbsp. **fresh basil**, chopped
- 1 tsp. **molasses**
- 1 piece **chicken** (4–6 oz.)

1. In a Ziploc bag, combine salt, pepper, Worcestershire sauce, vinegar, olive oil, honey, mustard, garlic, basil, and molasses. Seal bag and shake until contents are mixed thoroughly. Place chicken in Ziploc bag and marinate meat in the refrigerator for 1–2 hours.
2. Heat grill to medium-high. Grill chicken for 5 minutes on each side, until golden brown on both sides and no longer pink in the center.

Chicken Curry

- 1 Tbsp. butter
- 2 Tbsp. honey
- 1 Tbsp. **Dijon mustard**
- 1 tsp. curry powder
- dash of nutmeg
- dash of salt
- 1 cup water
- 1 piece **chicken** (4–6 oz.)
- ½ cup rice
- ½ tsp. butter
- pinch of salt

1. Preheat oven to 350 degrees. In a small saucepan, whisk together butter, honey, mustard, curry, nutmeg, and salt. Bring mixture to a boil, stirring constantly.
2. Grease a small baking dish and add chicken. Pour sauce mixture over the chicken. Cover with aluminum foil. Bake for about 35 minutes, until chicken is cooked through.
3. Meanwhile, bring 1 cup water to a boil in a small saucepan. Add rice, butter, and a pinch of salt. Bring back to a boil. Reduce heat to a simmer. Cover and let cook for 15–20 minutes. Fluff rice with a fork. Serve the chicken mixture over rice.

Chicken Enchiladas

- ¾ tsp. garlic powder
- ¾ tsp. cumin
- 1 **chicken breast**, boneless, skinless
- 2 tsp. olive oil
- ½ cup **yellow onion**, chopped
- ½ cup **mushrooms**, sliced
- ½ tsp. garlic, minced
- 1 cup **stewed tomatoes**
- ¾ tsp. chili powder (more if desired)
- ¼ cup **corn**
- ½ cup **cheddar cheese**, shredded
- 2 **tortillas**
- 2 Tbsp. **fresh cilantro**, diced

1. Preheat oven to 350 degrees. In a small bowl, mix ½ tsp. garlic powder and ½ tsp. cumin. Add chicken and fully coat.
2. Add 1 tsp. olive oil and chicken to a skillet on medium heat. Sauté chicken for 5–7 minutes on each side, until cooked through. Set aside to cool. Shred chicken by pulling apart with fingers or fork.
3. In the same skillet, add remaining olive oil, onion, mushrooms, and garlic. Sauté for 3–5 minutes over medium-low heat until tender.
4. Meanwhile, puree tomatoes in a blender or food processor. Separate sauce evenly into two small bowls.
5. Add one bowl of pureed tomatoes, ½ tsp. chili powder, and corn to the skillet with onions. Simmer for about 3 minutes. Add chicken and half of the cheese. Mix well and turn off heat.
6. In the other bowl of pureed tomatoes, add ¼ tsp. cumin, ¼ tsp. garlic powder, ¼ tsp. chili powder, and 2 Tbsp. water. Mix well. Dip tortilla in sauce. Place tortilla in skillet to cook for 1 minute on each side. Save extra mixture for later.
7. Grease a small bread baking dish and place tortilla inside. Add chicken mixture to the inside of each of the tortillas. Roll up each tortilla. Spread the rest of the sauce over the top of the tortillas. Sprinkle with remaining cheese.
8. Cover dish with aluminum foil and bake for 15–20 minutes. Garnish with cilantro.

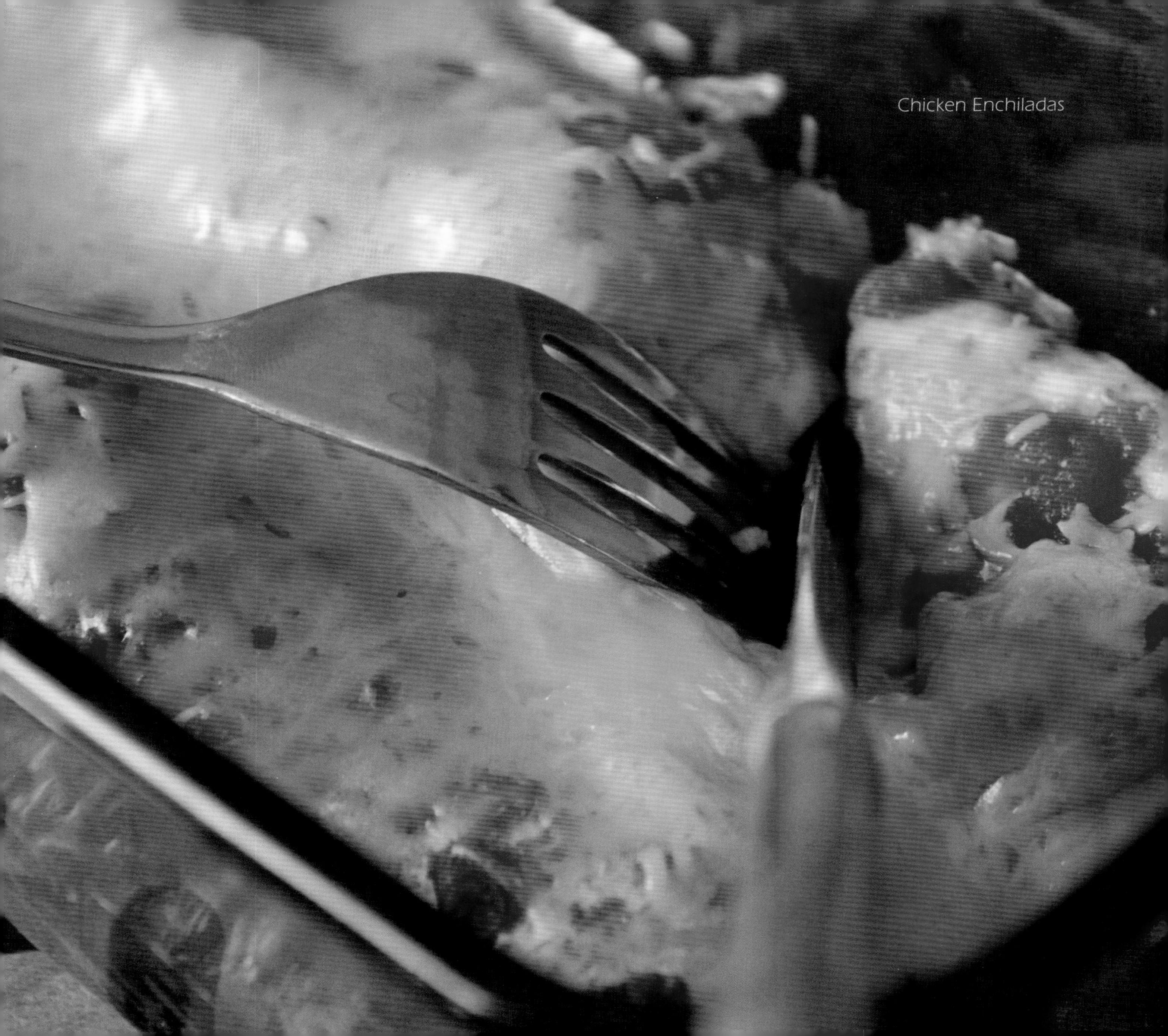

Chicken Enchiladas

Coconut Chicken

- ¼ cup. **plain yogurt**
- 2 tsp. olive oil
- ½ tsp. garlic, minced
- ⅛ tsp. of turmeric
- ¼ tsp. of garam masala
- ¼ tsp. cumin
- ½ tsp. salt
- 1 tsp. lemon juice
- 1 piece **chicken**, drumstick or thigh (4–6 oz.)
- ½ cup **yellow onion**, chopped
- ¼ cup **coconut milk**
- 1 Tbsp. **fresh cilantro**, chopped

1. In a small Ziploc bag, mix yogurt, 1 tsp. olive oil, garlic, turmeric, garam masala, cumin, salt, and lemon juice. Add chicken and marinate for 2–4 hours in the refrigerator (or preferably overnight).
2. Preheat oven to 375 degrees. Remove chicken from marinade. Set aside excess marinade. Add onions and the rest of the olive oil to a small skillet over medium-high heat. Cook for about 5 minutes, until tender. Add chicken to skillet. Sear chicken for about 4 minutes on each side.
3. Meanwhile, pour remaining marinade into a small saucepan and add coconut milk. Bring to a boil.
4. Place chicken and sauce in baking dish. Cover with aluminum foil, and bake for 30 minutes. Garnish with cilantro.

Citrus Chicken

- 1 piece **chicken** (4–6 oz.)
- dash of salt and ground pepper
- 1 Tbsp. **orange juice**
- 1 tsp. lemon juice
- 1 tsp. brown sugar
- 1 Tbsp. honey
- dash of cloves

1. Heat grill to medium-high. Season chicken with salt and pepper. Grill chicken breast for 5–7 minutes on each side, until golden brown on both sides and no longer pink in the center.
2. Meanwhile, in a small saucepan, whisk together orange juice, lemon juice, brown sugar, honey, and cloves. Bring mixture to a boil and keep at a boil, stirring constantly for 1–3 minutes or until syrupy. Apply glaze to finished meat.

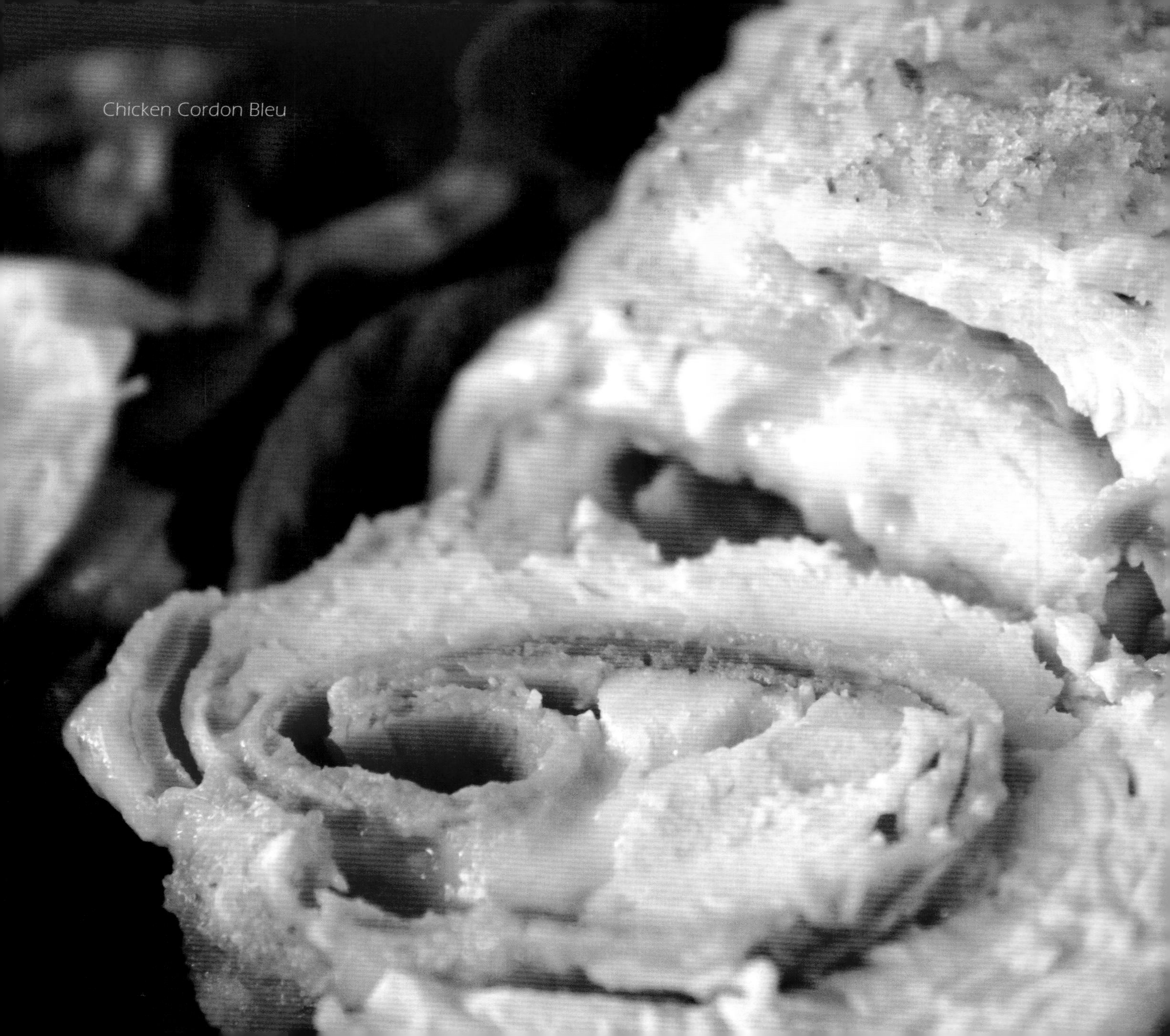

Chicken Cordon Bleu

Chicken Cordon Bleu

- 1 **chicken breast**, boneless, skinless
- 1–2 slices **Swiss cheese**
- 1–2 slices ham
- 2 Tbsp. **bread crumbs**
- 1 egg

1. Preheat oven to 400 degrees. Pound chicken until ½–¼ inch thick. Place cheese and ham on top of chicken. Roll all three and stick with a toothpick to keep from unrolling. Slice off just enough of ends to expose the circular roll.
2. Place bread crumbs in a small bowl. Whisk egg in another small bowl. Dip chicken roll in egg and then cover in bread crumb mixture.
3. Place chicken in greased baking dish. Cover with aluminum foil and place in oven. Bake for 30 minutes, or until there is no pink inside the chicken.

Grilled Cranberry Chicken

- 1 **chicken breast**, boneless, skinless
- coarse salt and ground pepper
- 2 Tbsp. cranberry sauce (with whole cranberries)
- 1 tsp. **orange juice**
- 1 tsp. honey
- 1 tsp. red wine vinegar

1. Heat grill to medium-high. Season chicken with salt and pepper. Grill chicken breast for 5 minutes on each side, until golden brown on both sides and no longer pink in the center.
2. Meanwhile, in a small saucepan, whisk together cranberry sauce, orange juice, honey, and red wine vinegar. Bring mixture to a boil and keep at a boil, stirring constantly for 1–3 minutes or until syrupy. Apply glaze to cooked meat.

Turkey Wrap

- 1 **tortilla** (whole grain recommended)
- 1 Tbsp. **cream cheese**
- 2–3 **slices turkey**
- 2–3 leaves **green leaf Romaine lettuce**
- 3–4 slices **avocado**
- 3–4 slices **tomato**

1. Spread cream cheese on one side of tortilla. Layer slices of turkey, lettuce, avocado, and tomato to cover entire tortilla.
2. Roll tortilla and hold together with toothpicks, if desired.

Honey Mustard Chicken

- 1 piece **chicken** (4–6 oz.)
- dash of salt and ground pepper
- 1 tsp. olive oil
- 1 Tbsp. **stone-ground mustard**
- 1 Tbsp. brown sugar
- 1 Tbsp. honey
- 1 tsp. white wine vinegar

1. Season chicken with salt and pepper. Add olive oil and chicken to a medium nonstick skillet. Sauté over medium heat for 5–7 minutes on each side, until chicken is golden on the outside and opaque throughout.
2. Meanwhile, in a small saucepan, whisk together mustard, brown sugar, honey, and white wine vinegar. Bring mixture to a boil. Reduce to a simmer, stirring constantly for 1–3 minutes or until syrupy. Apply glaze to finished meat.

Poppy Seed Chicken

- 1 cup **chicken breast**, cubed
- 2 Tbsp. **sour cream**
- 2 Tbsp. cream of chicken soup
- 1 tsp. melted butter
- 4–6 Ritz crackers or 2 Tbsp. **bread crumbs**
- ¼ tsp. poppy seeds

1. Preheat oven to 350 degrees. In a small bowl combine chicken, sour cream, and cream of chicken soup. Place mixture in a 3-inch ramekin.
2. In another small bowl, mix melted butter, crackers, and poppy seeds. Sprinkle on top of chicken mixture.
3. Place ramekin on a baking sheet and cover with aluminum foil. Bake for 25–30 minutes. Let cool for about 5 minutes.

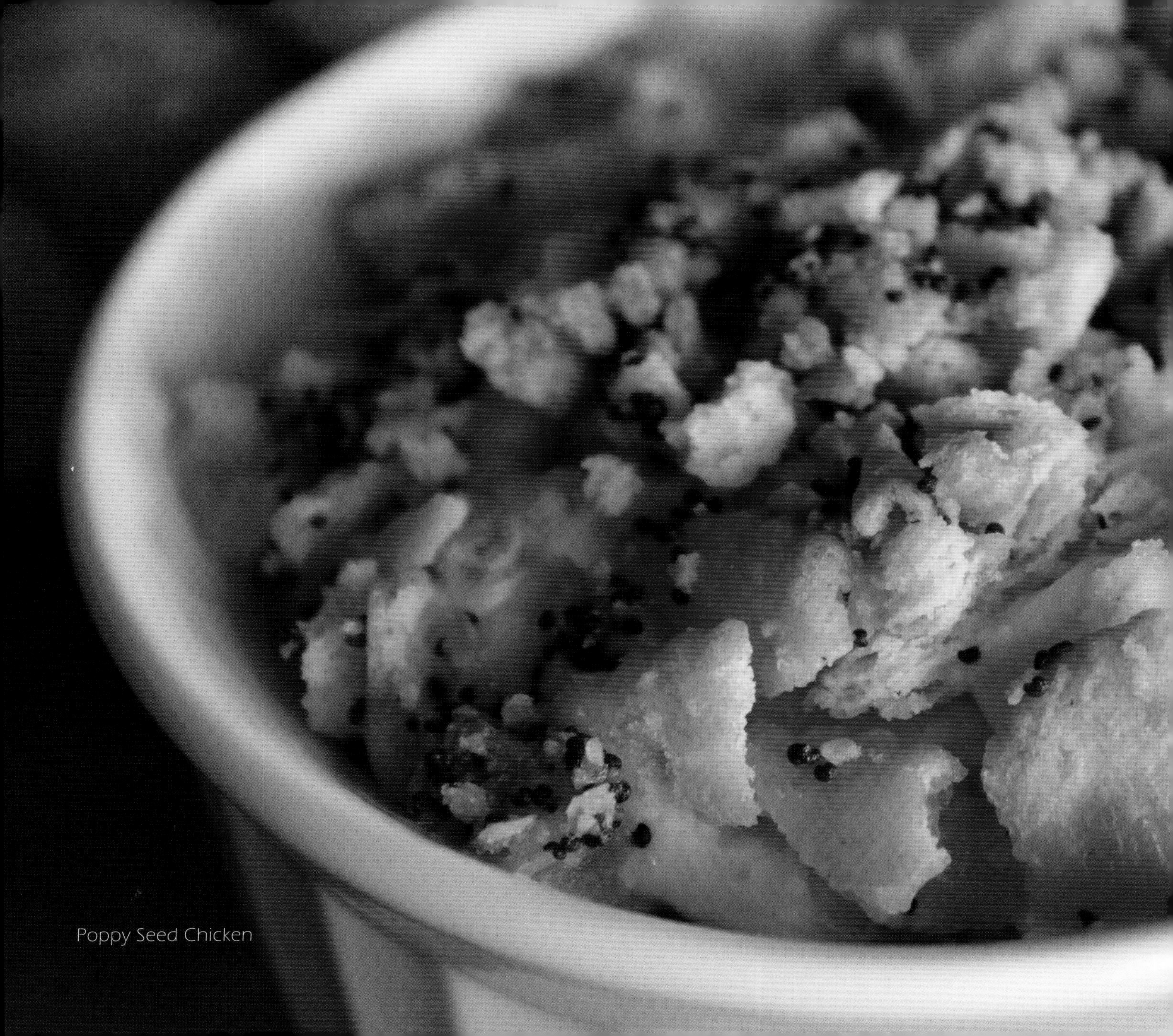

Poppy Seed Chicken

Marinara and Turkey Meatballs

- 3 oz. **ground turkey**
- ¼ tsp. garlic salt
- 1 tsp. whisked egg
- ¼ cup **yellow onion**, chopped
- 2 Tbsp. **celery**, chopped
- 2 Tbsp. **Romano cheese** (and extra for garnish)
- 2 tsp. **fresh parsley**, chopped
- dash of salt and pepper
- 2 Tbsp. **bread crumbs**
- 3–4 oz. dry spaghetti noodles
- 3 tsp. olive oil
- 1½ Tbsp. **tomato paste**
- ½ cup **stewed tomatoes**
- ¼ tsp. garlic, minced
- dash of oregano

1. In a small bowl, combine turkey, garlic salt, egg, half of the onion, half of the celery, cheese, ½ tsp. parsley, and a dash of salt and pepper. Shape into 3–4 meatballs. Coat meatballs with bread crumbs. Refrigerate for 15 minutes so the meatballs will hold their shape.
2. Meanwhile, fill a large pot with water and bring to a boil. Add spaghetti and cook for 5–10 minutes, until noodles are tender. Drain.
3. In a small skillet, add 1 tsp. olive oil and meatballs. Sauté for 10–15 minutes over medium heat. Make sure meatballs are evenly browned and cooked through. Remove from heat.
4. Add remaining onions to skillet and cook for 3–5 minutes, until tender. Set aside.
5. In a food processor or blender, add tomato paste, stewed tomatoes, 1 tsp. parsley, garlic, oregano, and a dash of salt and pepper. Add processed mixture to skillet with onions. Simmer for 5 minutes. Add meatballs and coat with sauce.
6. Transfer noodles to a plate. Add meatballs and sauce. Garnish with additional Romano cheese and parsley, if desired.

Raspberry Glazed Chicken

- 1 piece **chicken** (4–6 oz.)
- dash of salt and ground pepper
- 1½ tsp. olive oil
- 2 Tbsp. **raspberry preserves**
- 2 tsp. brown sugar
- 2 tsp. white wine vinegar

1. Season chicken with salt and pepper. In a medium nonstick skillet, heat olive oil over medium-high heat. Add chicken and sauté for 5–7 minutes on each side, until chicken is golden on the outside and opaque throughout.
2. Meanwhile, in a small saucepan, whisk together raspberry preserves, brown sugar, and white wine vinegar. Bring mixture to a boil. Reduce heat to a simmer, stirring constantly for 1–3 minutes or until syrupy. Apply to cooked meat.

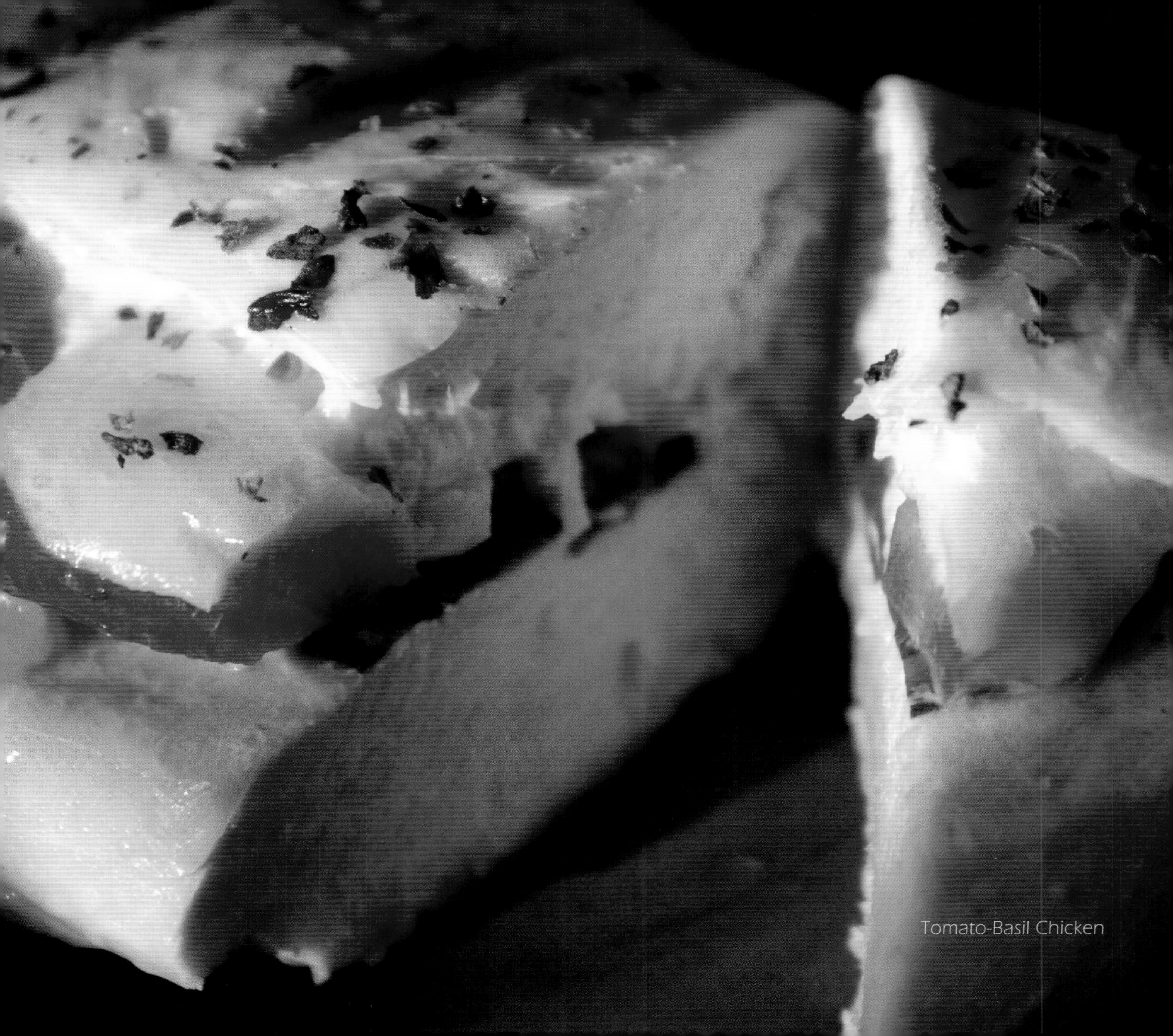

Tomato-Basil Chicken

Tomato-Basil Chicken

- 1 **chicken breast**, boneless, skinless
- 2–3 slices **mozzarella**
- 1 small **tomato**, thinly sliced
- 2–3 **fresh basil** leaves
- dash of salt and ground pepper
- dash of dried basil

1. Preheat oven to 375 degrees. Heat grill to medium-high heat. Sear each side of chicken for 2 minutes.
2. Cut a slit along the side of the chicken breast to create a pocket. Insert mozzarella, tomato, and basil into the chicken. Hold together with a toothpick if desired. Season with salt, pepper, and dried basil.
3. Place chicken in a greased baking dish. Cover with aluminum foil and bake for 20 minutes, or until there is no pink inside the chicken.

Sweet and Sour Chicken

- 1 egg, beaten
- ½ cup **chicken breast**, cubed
- 1 Tbsp. flour
- 1 Tbsp. cornstarch
- ⅛ tsp. garlic salt
- 1 cup water
- ½ cup rice
- ½ tsp. butter
- pinch of salt
- ¼ cup **green pepper**, diced
- 2 Tbsp. **green onion**, divided between white and green parts
- 1½ tsp. garlic, minced
- 1 tsp. vegetable oil
- 2 Tbsp. sugar
- 1 Tbsp. white wine vinegar
- 2 Tbsp. water
- 1 tsp. soy sauce
- 1 tsp. **ketchup**
- 1½ tsp. cornstarch

1. Dip chicken cubes in beaten egg. In a Ziploc bag, mix flour, cornstarch, and garlic salt. Place chicken in the bag with flour mixture and shake to coat completely.
2. Bring 1 cup of water to a boil in a small saucepan. Add rice, butter, and a pinch of salt. Bring to a boil again. Reduce heat to a simmer. Cover and let cook for 15–20 minutes. Fluff rice with a fork.
3. Add vegetable oil to a small skillet and add coated chicken, green peppers, white parts of the green onion, and garlic. Sauté over medium heat for about 5 minutes. Mix often to make sure chicken cooks evenly. It should be a light golden brown.
4. Meanwhile, in a small bowl, mix the sugar, white wine vinegar, water, soy sauce, ketchup, and cornstarch. Add mixture to chicken in the skillet and cook for 2 minutes. The mixture will thicken instantly. Mix chicken and sauce well.
5. Serve chicken mixture over rice. Garnish with green parts of the green onion.

Apricot Chicken

- 1 **chicken breast**, boneless, skinless
- 1 **dried apricot**
- 2 **fresh mint** leaves (extra for garnish)
- 1 tsp. whisked egg
- 1 Tbsp. **bread crumbs**
- 2 Tbsp. apricot preserves
- 2 tsp. brown sugar
- 1 pinch cloves

1. Preheat oven to 375 degrees. Place chicken in a greased baking dish. Cut a slit along the side of the chicken breast to create a pocket. Stuff with apricot and mint leaves. Hold together with a toothpick if needed. Brush on egg. Sprinkle bread crumbs over chicken. Cover dish with aluminum foil. Bake for 20–25 minutes.
2. When chicken is about 5 minutes from being done, whisk together apricot preserves, brown sugar, and cloves in a small saucepan. Bring mixture to a boil and then stir constantly for one minute. Reduce heat and let simmer for about 5 minutes. Drizzle glaze over finished chicken. Garnish with extra mint leaves.

Teriyaki Chicken

- 3 Tbsp. soy sauce
- 1 ½ tsp. rice vinegar
- ¾ tsp. sesame oil
- 2 Tbsp. white sugar
- ¼ tsp. **fresh ginger**, minced
- 1 **chicken breast**, boneless, skinless
- 1 tsp. garlic, minced
- ½ cup rice
- ½ tsp. butter
- pinch of salt
- ¼ tsp. cornstarch
- ¼ tsp. **sesame seeds**

1. In a small saucepan over medium-high heat, add soy sauce, rice vinegar, sesame oil, sugar, and ginger. Bring to a boil. Allow sauce to sit for a few minutes to cool. Slice raw chicken lengthwise. Add chicken to a Ziploc bag with sauce. Marinate for 1–2 hours.
2. Remove chicken from marinade and reserve the excess marinade to use as a sauce.
3. Heat grill to medium-high. Grill chicken breast slices for 3–5 minutes on each side, until no longer pink in the center.
4. Bring 1 cup water to a boil in a small saucepan. Add rice, butter, and a pinch of salt. Bring to a boil again. Reduce heat to a simmer. Cover and cook for 15–20 minutes. Fluff rice with a fork.
5. Meanwhile, in another small saucepan, bring excess marinade to a boil. Add cornstarch and mix well until sauce is thicker. Serve chicken mixture over rice. Drizzle with sauce and garnish with sesame seeds.

Teriyaki Chicken

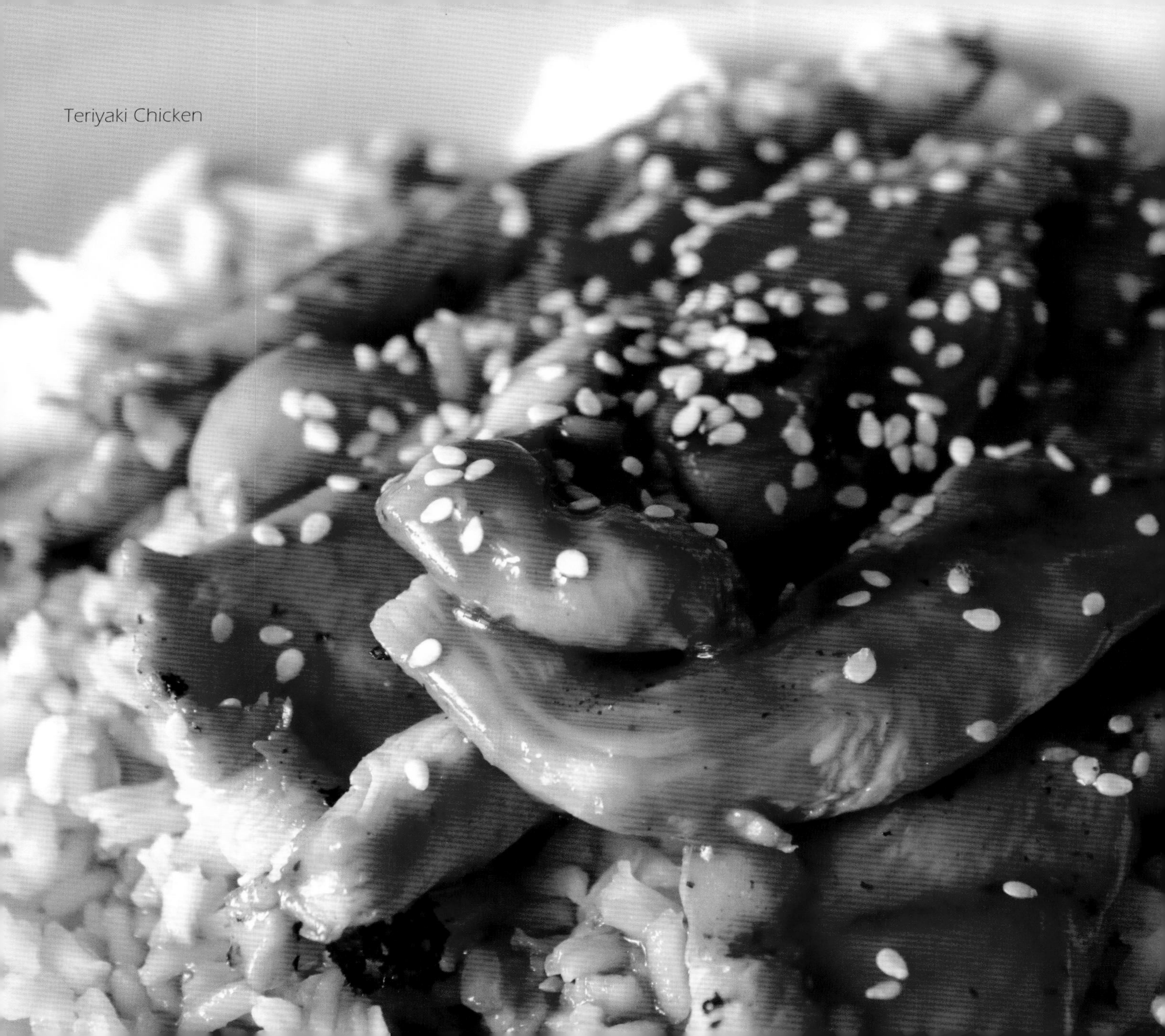

Turkey Dumplings

Filling

- 1 **asparagus stock**, chopped
- 1 tsp. sesame seed oil
- ¼ tsp. fresh ginger, minced
- ¼ tsp. garlic, minced
- 1 Tbsp. **green onions**, chopped
- ½ tsp. soy sauce
- 2 Tbsp. **ground turkey**

- 6 wonton wraps
- 1 Tbsp. rice vinegar
- 2 Tbsp. soy sauce
- 1 tsp. sesame seed oil
- 1 tsp. **green onions**, thinly chopped

1. In a food processor or blender, combine asparagus, sesame oil, ginger, garlic, green onions, and soy sauce. Mix well. Remove from food processor and stir in ground turkey.
2. Fill each wonton wrapper with 1 tsp. turkey mixture. Brush edges of wonton wrap with water. Fold wrap diagonally to make a triangle, and press edges together and twist.
3. Place steamer rack in a pot. Fill pot half full of water. Arrange dumplings so they are not touching. Steam for 15 minutes.
4. Meanwhile, in a small serving bowl, combine rice vinegar, soy sauce, sesame seed oil, and green onions for dipping sauce.

Mango Chicken

- 1 **chicken breast**, boneless, skinless
- 1 **mango**, julienne
- 2–3 slices **mozzarella cheese**
- 1 ½ Tbsp. **pineapple juice**
- 1 tsp. brown sugar
- ½ tsp. white wine vinegar
- 1 Tbsp. **fresh cilantro** leaves, chopped

1. Preheat oven to 375 degrees. Place chicken in a greased baking dish. Cut a slit along the side of the chicken breast to create a pocket. Stuff with mango and mozzarella. Hold together with a toothpick if needed. Cover dish with aluminum foil. Bake for 20–25 minutes.
2. Meanwhile, in a small saucepan, bring pineapple juice, brown sugar, and vinegar to a boil. Reduce heat to a simmer until chicken is done cooking. Transfer chicken to a serving plate. Drizzle glaze over chicken. Garnish with cilantro.

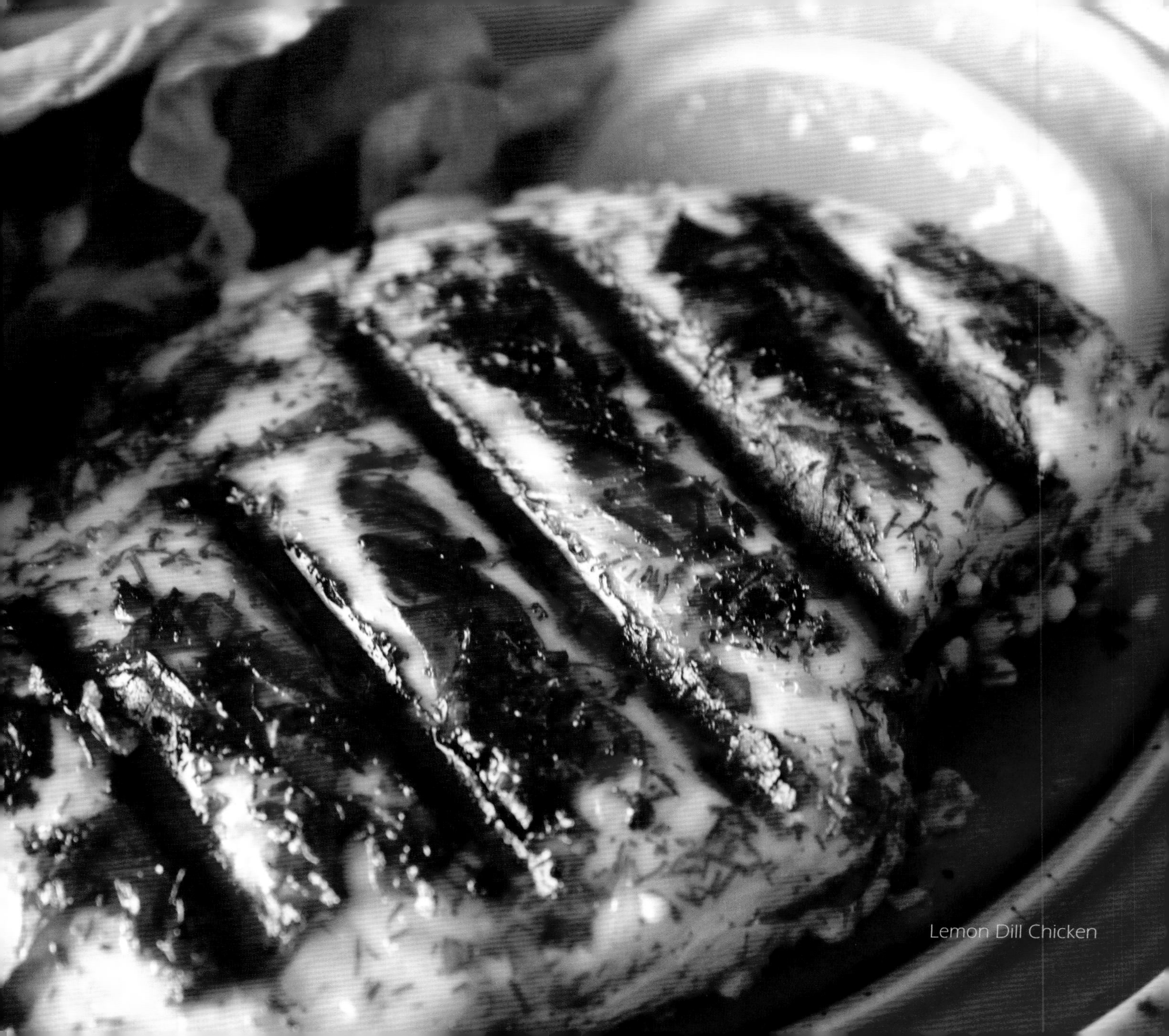

Lemon Dill Chicken

Lemon Dill Chicken

- dash of salt and pepper
- 1 Tbsp. olive oil
- 1 Tbsp. **fresh mint** leaves, chopped
- 1 Tbsp. **fresh basil** leaves, chopped
- ½ tsp. garlic clove minced
- 1 ½ tsp. lemon juice
- ½ tsp. **lemon zest**
- ½ tsp. dill weed
- 1 tsp. sugar
- ¼ tsp. oregano
- 1 tsp. white wine vinegar
- 1 piece **chicken** (4–6 oz.)

1. In a Ziploc bag, combine salt, pepper, olive oil, mint, basil, garlic, lemon juice, lemon zest, dill weed, sugar, oregano, and white wine vinegar. Seal bag and shake until contents are mixed thoroughly. Place chicken in Ziploc bag and marinate in refrigerator for 2–4 hours (depending on how much flavor you want).
2. Heat grill to medium-high. Grill chicken breast 5–10 minutes on each side, until no longer pink in the center.

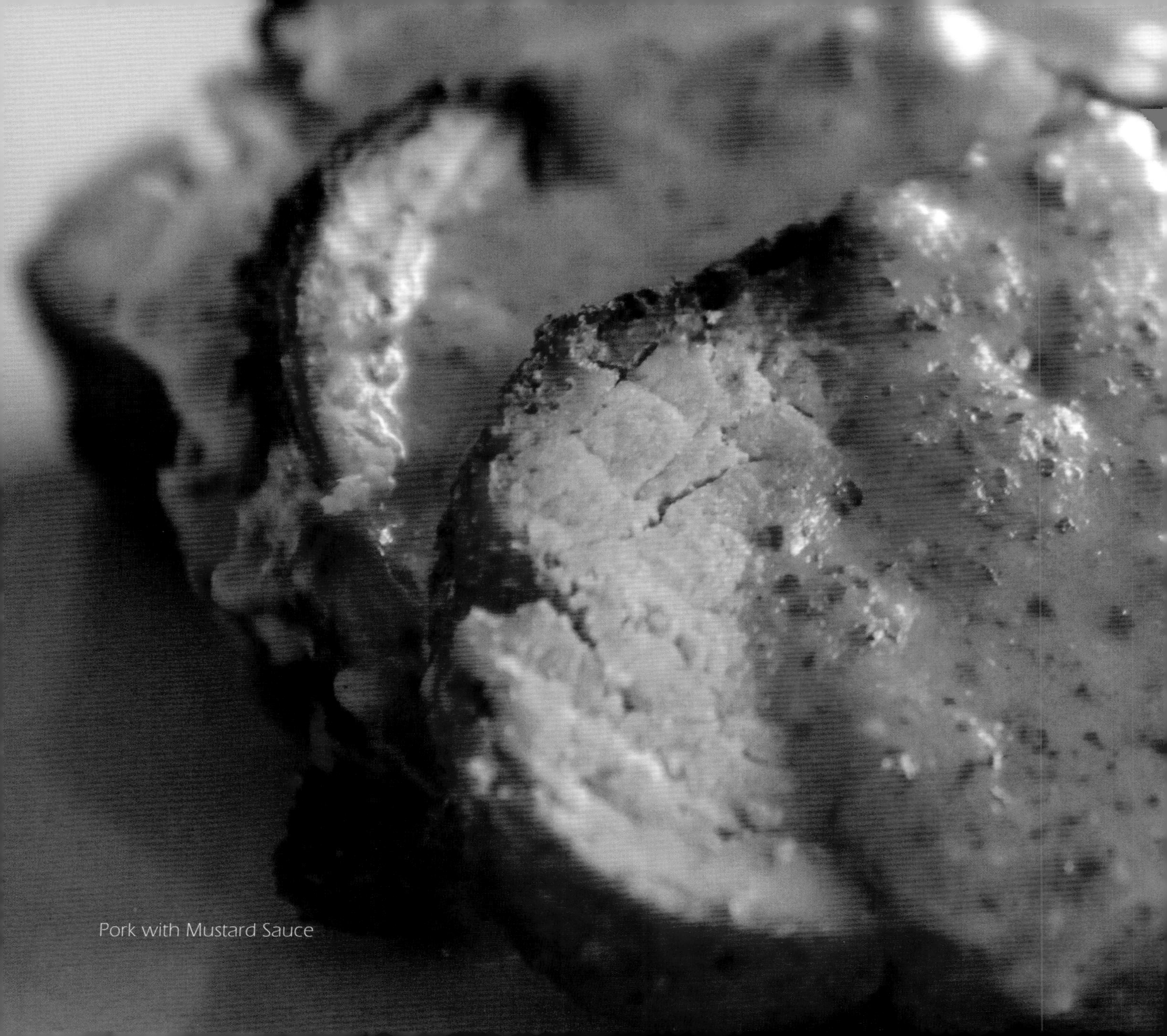

Pork with Mustard Sauce

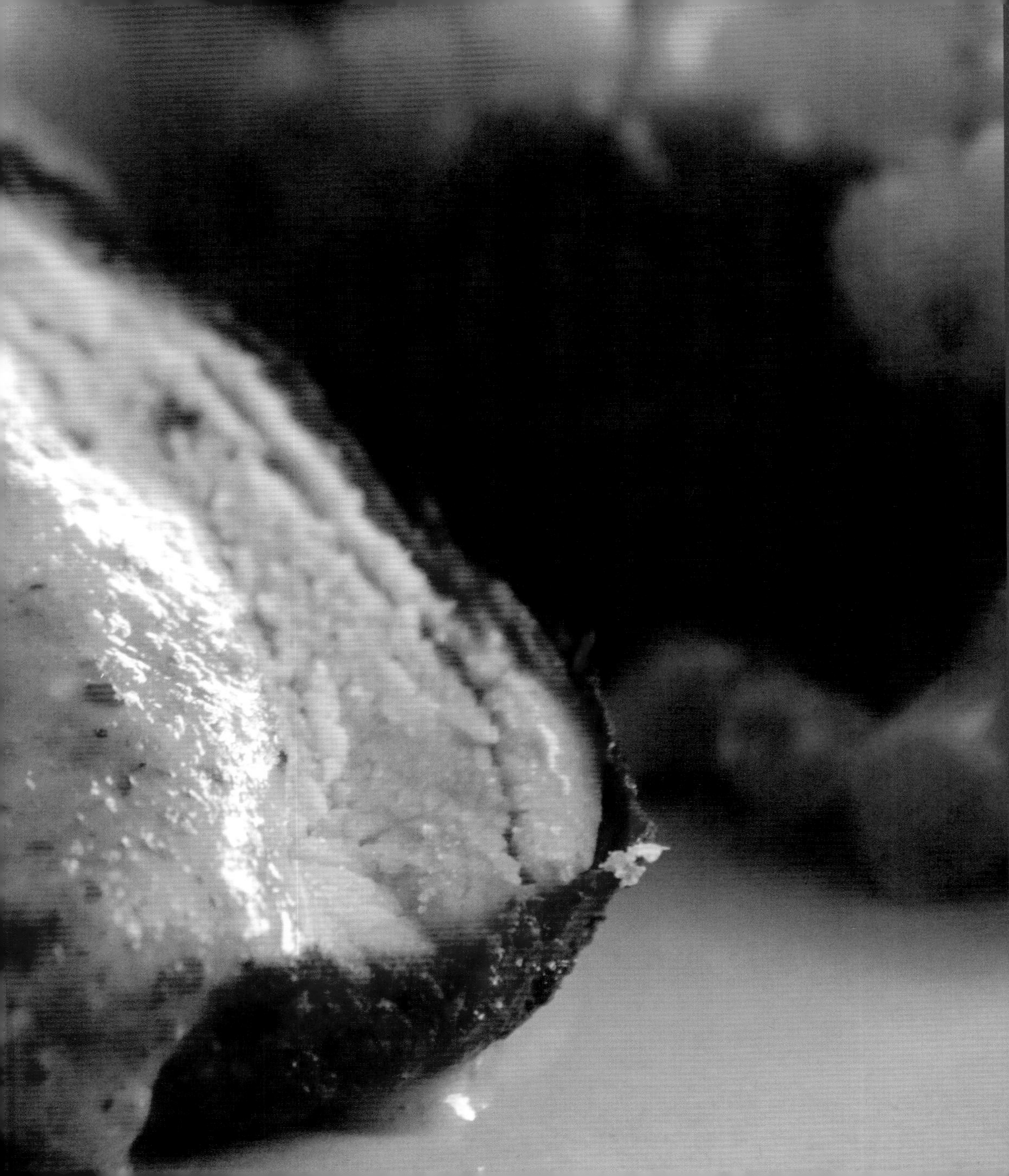

Red Meat

Red Meat

Red meat is an American household staple. Slogans like "Beef: It's what's for dinner" have been ingrained into our culture. So if it's what's for dinner, making sure that we have good recipes tailored to a serving size for one will keep us healthy and happy. Several types of meat fit into the red meat category, but in this cookbook we are only going to focus on pork and beef because they are the most affordable and accessible types of red meat.

Beef

Beef is quite versatile and is used in many dishes. Let's review the basic regions of the cow that the different cuts of beef are taken from. There are a few recipes that specify the type of beef needed. Recipes that don't specify the cut are usually referring to loin or rib-eye beef, which is also known as steak.

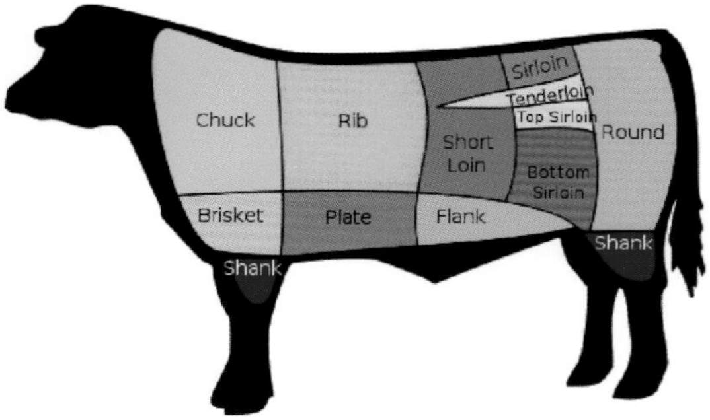

Additionally, I thought it would be helpful to review what has come to be known as the thumb test for cooking or grilling steak. The thumb test assesses meat for tenderness and is a simple way of telling if your meat is cooked to your liking.

The Thumb Test

- **Rare**—Press your left thumb and forefinger (pointer finger) together like you're giving someone the "OK" signal. With the thumb and forefinger of your right hand, pinch the fleshy part of your left hand between the thumb and forefinger. This is how rare steak feels to the touch. It should feel soft and bouncy. The core temperature should be 125 degrees.
- **Medium**—Press your left thumb and middle finger together and with your right hand, pinch the fleshy part between your thumb and forefinger. This is what medium steak feels like. You should feel some give. The core temperature should be 140 degrees.
- **Well Done**—Press your left thumb and little finger together and with your right hand, pinch the fleshy part between your thumb and forefinger. This is what a well done steak feels like. It is firm, with little give. The core temperature should be 160 degrees.

Pork

The part of the pig that most of your cuts will come from is the loin. From the loin you get the following cuts of pork: roasts (blade loin roast, center loin roast, sirloin roast), back ribs (baby back ribs, riblets), bacon, pork cutlets, and pork chops. In this cookbook, there are recipes for two different cuts of pork: pork chops and pork tenderloin. Both of these choices are usually quite common in the grocery store.

However, to learn a little more about what part of the pig each cut comes from, refer to this diagram.

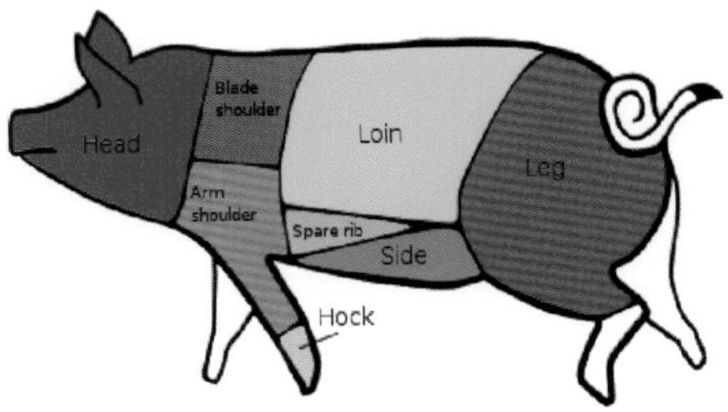

French Dip Sandwich

- 1 (6-inch) portion of **French baguette**
- 2 slices of **provolone** or **Swiss cheese**
- 4–6 oz. **roast beef**
- 2 tsp. au jus gravy mix
- 1 cup water

1. Broil French baguette in oven for 1–2 minutes. Watch so it doesn't burn.
2. If you would like the cheese melted, pull bread out of the oven and add cheese on top of the bread. Place back in the oven for about 2 minutes.
3. Remove bread from the oven and add cheese (if not already added) and roast beef to the sandwich.
4. Meanwhile, add au jus mix and water to a small pot. Bring to a boil. Place in a small serving bowl or cup. Transfer sandwich and small serving bowl to a plate.

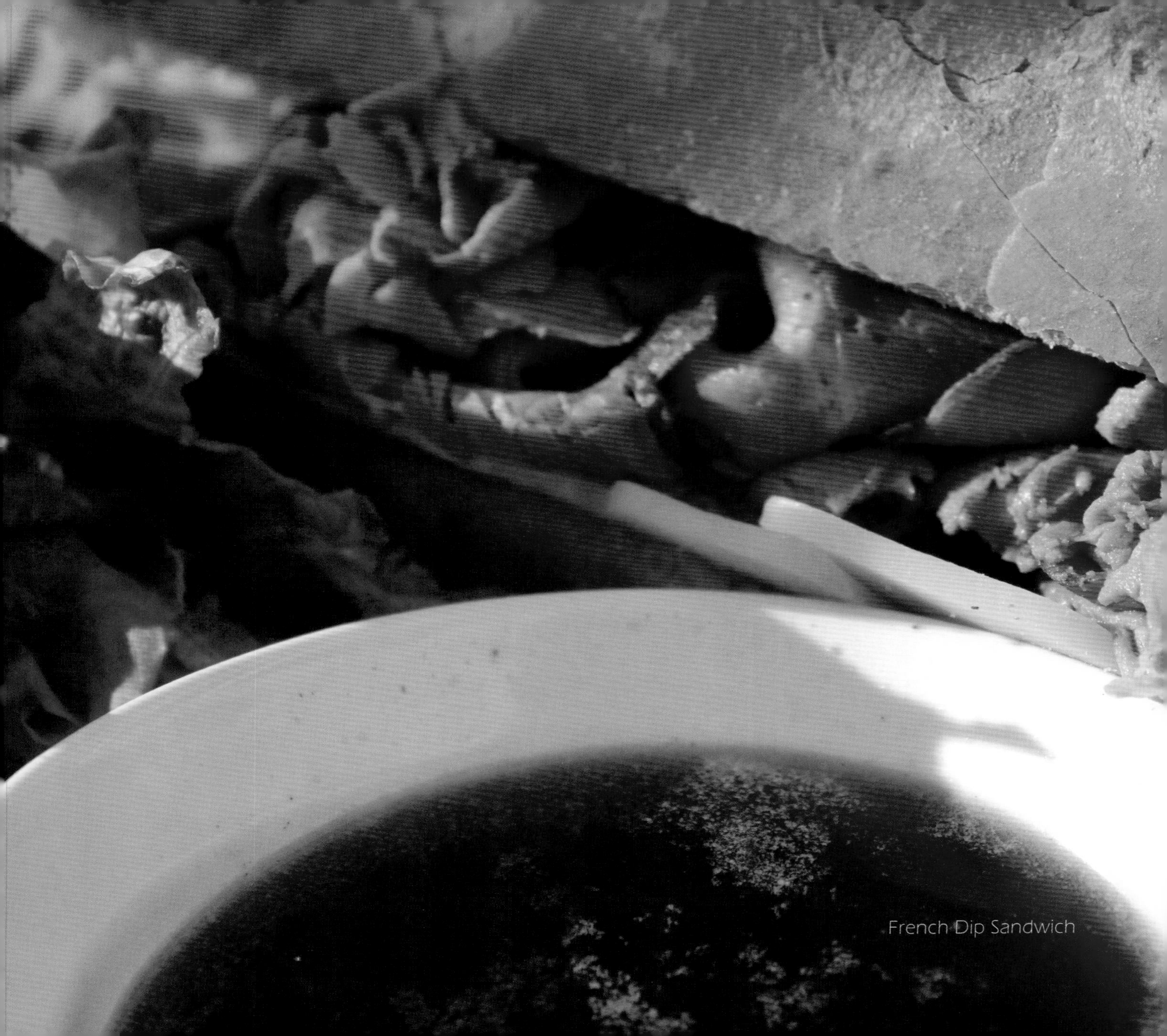
French Dip Sandwich

Apple Cider Steak

- 2 Tbsp. **apple cider**
- 1 Tbsp. cider vinegar
- 1 tsp. white wine (or white grape juice)
- 1 Tbsp. olive oil
- 1 tsp. honey
- ½ tsp. garlic, minced
- 1 Tbsp. **apple**, mashed (extra slices for garnish)
- dash of salt and pepper
- 4–6 oz. **beef sirloin/ steak**

1. In a small saucepan, combine apple cider, cider vinegar, white wine, olive oil, honey, garlic, mashed apple, salt, and pepper to make the marinade. Bring to a boil. Remove from heat.
2. Place meat and warm marinade in a Ziploc bag and coat thoroughly. Marinate in the refrigerator for 2–4 hours.
3. Heat grill to medium-high heat. Grill steak for 2–5 minutes on each side, depending on how you like your steak. (Use the thumb test on page 77 to determine tenderness.)
4. Transfer meat to a plate. Garnish with extra sliced apple.

BBQ Steak

- 1 Tbsp. **ketchup**
- ¾ tsp. brown sugar
- ¾ tsp. **Worcestershire sauce**
- ½ tsp. apple cider vinegar
- ¼ tsp. **molasses**
- 1/8 tsp. garlic powder
- ½ tsp. **stone-ground mustard**
- dash of salt and pepper
- 4–6 oz. **beef sirloin/steak**

1. In a small saucepan, bring ketchup, brown sugar, Worcestershire sauce, vinegar, molasses, garlic powder, mustard, salt, and pepper to a boil. Let simmer for 5 minutes. Reserve half of sauce for serving. Coat steak in remaining sauce.
2. Heat grill to medium-high heat. Grill steak for 2–5 minutes on each side, depending on how you like your steak. (Use the thumb test on page 77 to determine tenderness.)
3. Transfer meat to a plate. Apply extra sauce as desired.

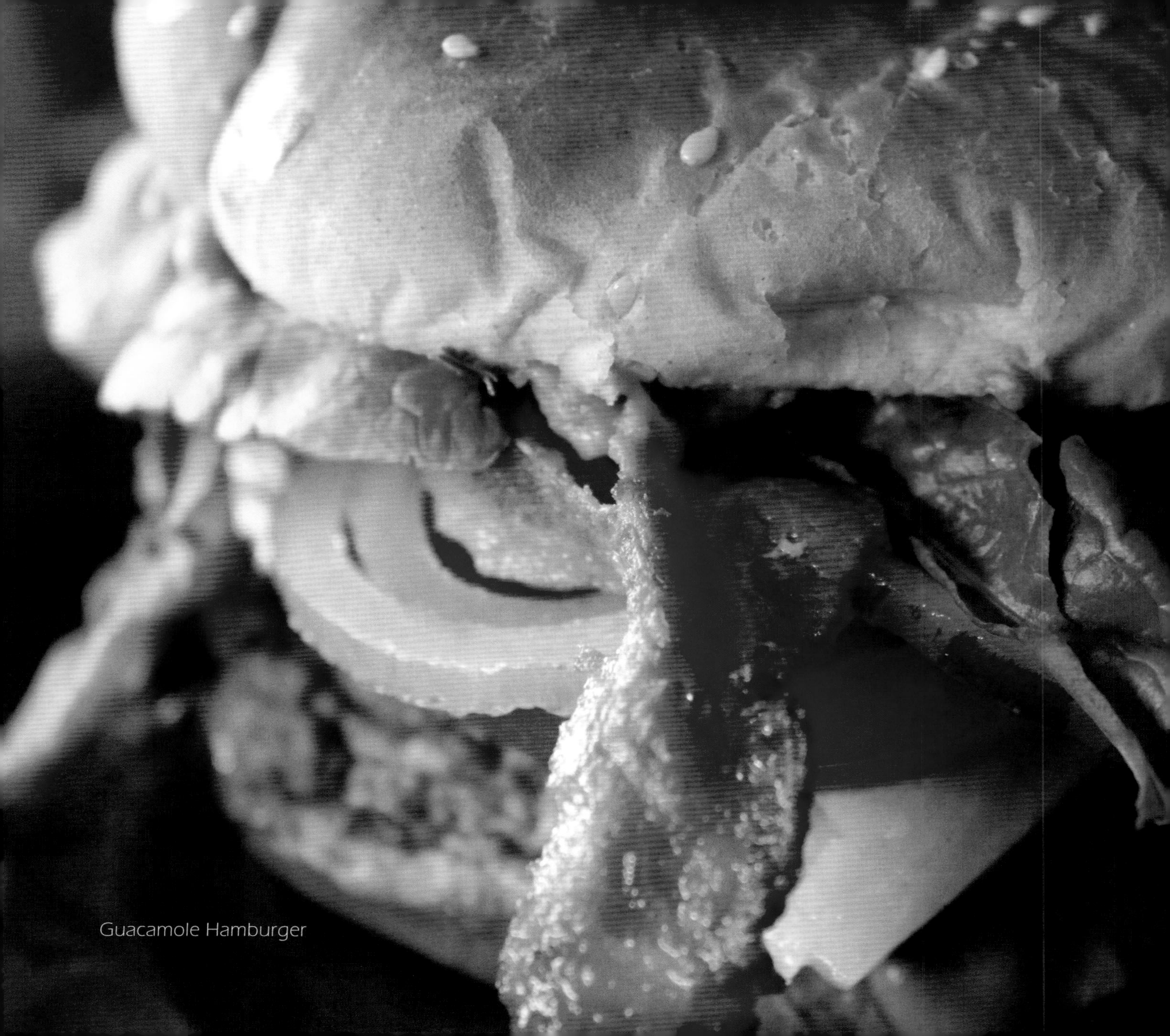

Guacamole Hamburger

Guacamole Hamburger

- 4–6 oz. **ground beef**
- dash of salt and ground pepper
- 2 tsp. **Worcestershire sauce**
- 1 slice of Monterey Jack cheese
- 1 **hamburger bun**
- 2 slices **bacon**
- 2–3 leaves of **red leaf Romaine lettuce**
- 1 **tomato**, sliced
- 1–2 slices of **red onion**
- 2–3 Tbsp. **guacamole**

1. Season ground beef with salt and pepper and Worcestershire sauce. Shape into patty. Grill over medium-high heat. Cook for about 3–7 minutes on each side, depending on how well done you want your burger. Add cheese on top of meat for the last 2 minutes. Toast bun on grill as well, 1–2 minutes on each side.
2. In a small skillet, cook bacon for 2 minutes on each side over medium heat. Pat down bacon to remove extra grease.
3. Build the burger by placing the meat and cheese on the bottom half of the bun and then layering lettuce, tomato, onion, bacon, and guacamole.

Beef Bulgogi

Marinade

- 1 tsp. **sesame seeds**, toasted
- 1 tsp. toasted sesame oil
- 1 tsp. rice vinegar
- 1 tsp. peanut oil
- ½ tsp. soy sauce
- ½ tsp. brown sugar
- ½ tsp. garlic, minced
- dash of salt and pepper

Beef Mixture

- 3–4 oz **beef sirloin**, thinly sliced diagonally
- ½ cup **red onion**, sliced
- ½ **carrot**, julienne
- ½ cup **green bell pepper**, chopped
- ½ Tbsp. vegetable oil
- 2 **green onions**, chopped
- ¼ tsp. **lime juice**

1. In a Ziploc bag, combine marinade ingredients. Slice beef diagonally into strips. Add beef, red onion, carrot, and bell peppers to bag. Coat well and marinate in the refrigerator for 1 hour.
2. In a medium skillet, add vegetable oil, green onion, and bell pepper. Sauté for 5–7 minutes over medium-low heat until tender. Remove from heat.
3. Meanwhile, turn on oven broiler and line baking sheet with aluminum foil. Arrange beef slices on baking sheet so they're not overlapping. Broil for 4–6 minutes on each side, basting with the rest of the marinade.
4. Add meat to skillet with vegetables. Add lime juice and green onion and mix well. Transfer to a plate. Garnish with extra sesame seeds.

Honey Lemon Pork Chops

- 2 tsp. olive oil
- ½ tsp. garlic, minced
- 1 tsp. apple cider vinegar
- 1½ tsp. lemon juice
- ½ tsp. **lemon zest**
- 1 Tbsp. honey
- 1 tsp. **fresh basil**, chopped
- 1 tsp. thyme
- pinch of salt and pepper
- 1 **pork chop** (about 4–6 oz.)

1. In a Ziploc bag, combine olive oil, garlic, apple cider vinegar, lemon juice, lemon zest, honey, basil, thyme, salt, and pepper. Seal the bag, and shake until contents are mixed thoroughly. Place pork chop in Ziploc bag and marinate for 1–2 hours.
2. Heat grill to medium-high heat. Cook pork chop for 3–5 minutes on each side. Transfer to a plate.

Pomegranate Glazed Pork

- ½ tsp. coriander
- ½ tsp. cumin
- pinch of cinnamon
- pinch of salt and pepper
- 4–6 oz. **pork tenderloin**
- 3 Tbsp. **pomegranate juice**
- 2 tsp. red wine vinegar
- ½ tsp. **molasses**
- ¼ tsp. rosemary
- ½ tsp. cornstarch

1. In a small bowl, combine coriander, cumin, cinnamon, salt, and pepper. Add pork to bowl and coat thoroughly.
2. Heat broiler. Line baking sheet with aluminum foil. Place pork on baking sheet about 4 inches from the top of the oven. Broil for 20–25 minutes, or until pork is cooked through.
3. Meanwhile, in a small saucepan over medium-high heat, combine pomegranate juice, vinegar, molasses, and rosemary. Bring to a boil, stirring constantly. Reduce heat. Add cornstarch and stir until mixture is thick. Remove from heat.
4. Transfer pork to a plate and slice. Drizzle with pomegranate glaze.

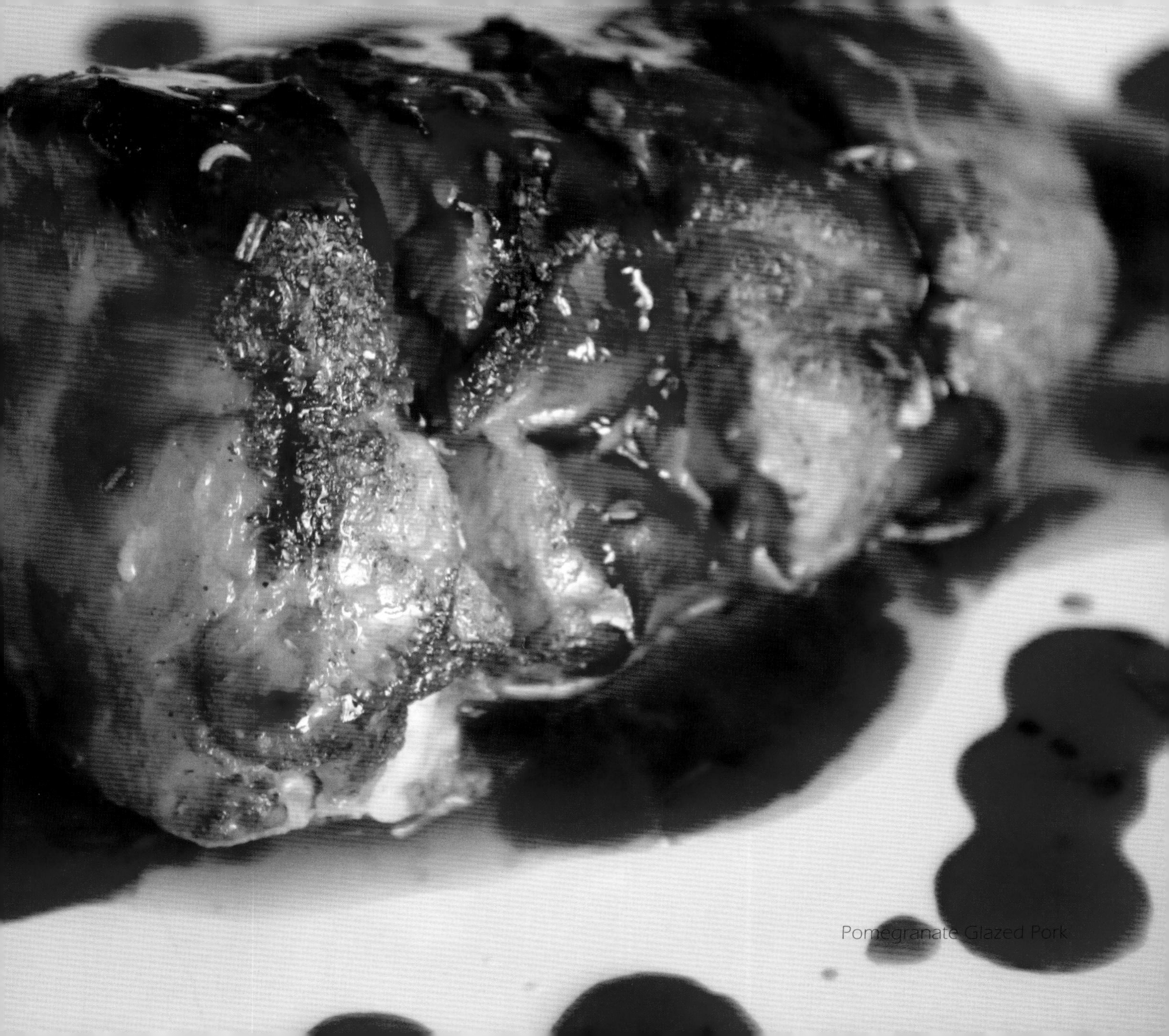

Pomegranate Glazed Pork

Pork with Mustard Sauce

- ½ tsp. coriander
- ¼ tsp. cinnamon
- dash of salt and pepper
- 4–6 oz. **pork tenderloin**
- 1 Tbsp. **stone-ground mustard**
- 1 Tbsp. **plain yogurt**
- 1 Tbsp. brown sugar
- dash of cloves

1. In a small bowl, combine coriander, cinnamon, salt, and pepper. Add pork to bowl and rub spices into meat thoroughly.
2. Turn on oven broiler and line baking sheet with aluminum foil. Lay pork on baking sheet and place on a rack about 4 inches from the top of the oven. Broil for 20–25 minutes, or until pork is cooked through.
3. Meanwhile, in a small saucepan, combine stone-ground mustard, yogurt, brown sugar, and cloves. Bring to a boil and stir for one minute. Remove from heat.
4. Transfer pork to a plate and slice. Drizzle with mustard sauce.

Pork Quesadilla

- 2 **tortillas** (whole grain recommended)
- ¼ lb. shredded pork
- 2 Tbsp. barbecue sauce
- 1 cup **cheddar cheese**, shredded
- 2 Tbsp. **green onions**, chopped
- 1 Tbsp. butter
- 2 Tbsp. **sour cream**
- 2 Tbsp. **fresh cilantro**, chopped

1. Fold both tortillas in half. Fill tortillas with even amounts of shredded pork, BBQ sauce, cheese, and onions.
2. Melt butter in a medium skillet. Add one tortilla at a time. Cook quesadilla for 2–3 minutes on each side.
3. Cut tortilla into three triangles and garnish with sour cream and cilantro.

Strawberry Pork Chops

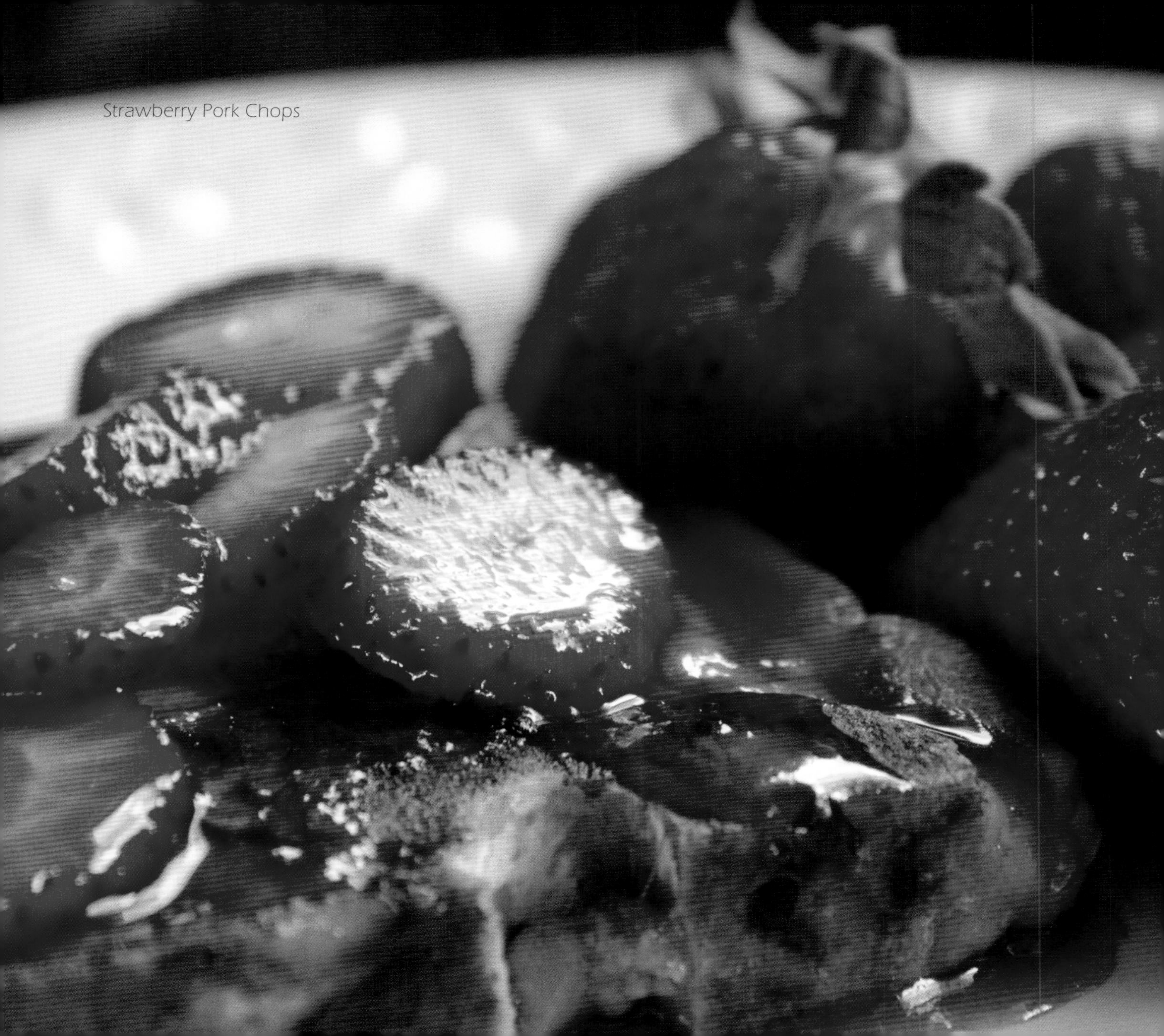

Strawberry Pork Chops

- 1 **pork chop** (about 4–6 oz.)
- dash of salt and ground pepper
- 2 Tbsp. strawberry preserves
- 2 tsp. brown sugar
- 2 tsp. white wine vinegar
- 2 **fresh strawberries**, sliced (extra for garnish)

1. Heat grill to medium-high heat. Season pork with salt and pepper. Place pork on grill. Cook for 4–6 minutes on each side, or until cooked through. Place pork on a plate.
2. In a small saucepan, whisk together strawberry preserves, brown sugar, white wine vinegar, and strawberries. Bring mixture to a boil and keep at a boil, stirring constantly for 1–3 minutes or until syrupy. Drizzle over cooked meat. Garnish with fresh strawberries.

Sweet and Spicy Pork Chops

- ½ tsp. cinnamon
- 1 ½ tsp. brown sugar
- ½ tsp. cumin
- ½ tsp. cardamom
- pinch of nutmeg
- pinch of cloves
- ½ tsp. salt
- pinch of pepper
- 1 **pork chop** (about 4–6 oz.)
- 1 tsp. olive oil

1. In a small bowl, combine cinnamon, brown sugar, cumin, cardamom, cloves, nutmeg, salt, and pepper. Rub into meat.
2. Heat olive oil in a small skillet. Place pork in skillet. Sauté for 4–5 minutes on each side, or until cooked through.

Steak Fajitas

- 1 tsp. vegetable oil
- ½ of a **yellow onion**, sliced in circles
- ½ of a **green bell pepper**, julienne
- ½ of a **yellow bell pepper**, julienne
- ½ of a **red bell pepper**, julienne
- 4–6 oz. flank or skirt steak, sliced diagonally
- 2 **tortillas** (whole grain recommended)
- 1–2 Tbsp. **guacamole**
- 1–2 Tbsp. **sour cream**
- 2 tsp. **fresh cilantro**, chopped

Marinade

- ½ tsp. **lime juice**
- 1 tsp. of olive oil
- ½ tsp. garlic, minced
- ¼ tsp. ground cumin
- ¼ tsp. chili powder

1. In a Ziploc bag, combine marinade ingredients. Add meat to bag, coat well, and refrigerate 1 hour.
2. In a medium skillet, add vegetable oil, onion, and bell peppers. Sauté for 3–5 minutes over medium-low heat until vegetables are tender. Remove from heat.
3. Meanwhile, heat broiler and line baking sheet with aluminum foil. Arrange beef slices on baking sheet so they are not overlapping. Broil for 4–6 minutes on each side. Baste with the rest of the marinade.
4. Add meat to skillet with vegetables and mix well.
5. On a plate, assemble fajitas by starting with the tortilla (it's better warm) and then adding meat mixture, guacamole, sour cream, and cilantro.

Beef Stir Fry

- 1 cup water
- ½ cup rice
- ½ tsp. butter
- pinch of salt
- 2 tsp. olive oil
- ¼ cup **yellow onion**, chopped
- ½ **red pepper**, julienne
- ½ **green pepper**, julienne
- ½ **yellow pepper**, julienne
- 5–7 snap peas
- 1 tsp. garlic, minced
- 3 oz. **stir fry beef**
- 2 Tbsp. soy sauce
- ½ tsp. garlic powder
- ¼ tsp. ground ginger
- ¼ tsp. flour

1. Bring 1 cup water to a boil in a small saucepan. Add rice, butter, and a pinch of salt. Bring to a boil again. Reduce heat to a simmer. Cover and let cook for 15–20 minutes. Fluff rice with a fork.
2. While rice is cooking, heat 1 tsp. olive oil in a medium skillet. Add onions and sauté over medium-low heat for 5–7 minutes, or until soft. Add peppers, snap peas, and garlic. Sauté for 10 more minutes, stirring occasionally.
3. Add meat and 1 more tsp. olive oil. Cook for 7–10 minutes, until meat is cooked through and vegetables are soft.
4. Meanwhile, in a small bowl, combine soy sauce, garlic powder, ground ginger, and flour. Add meat to vegetable mixture in skillet and let cook 1 minute.
5. Dish rice onto a plate and top with the meat and vegetable mixture.

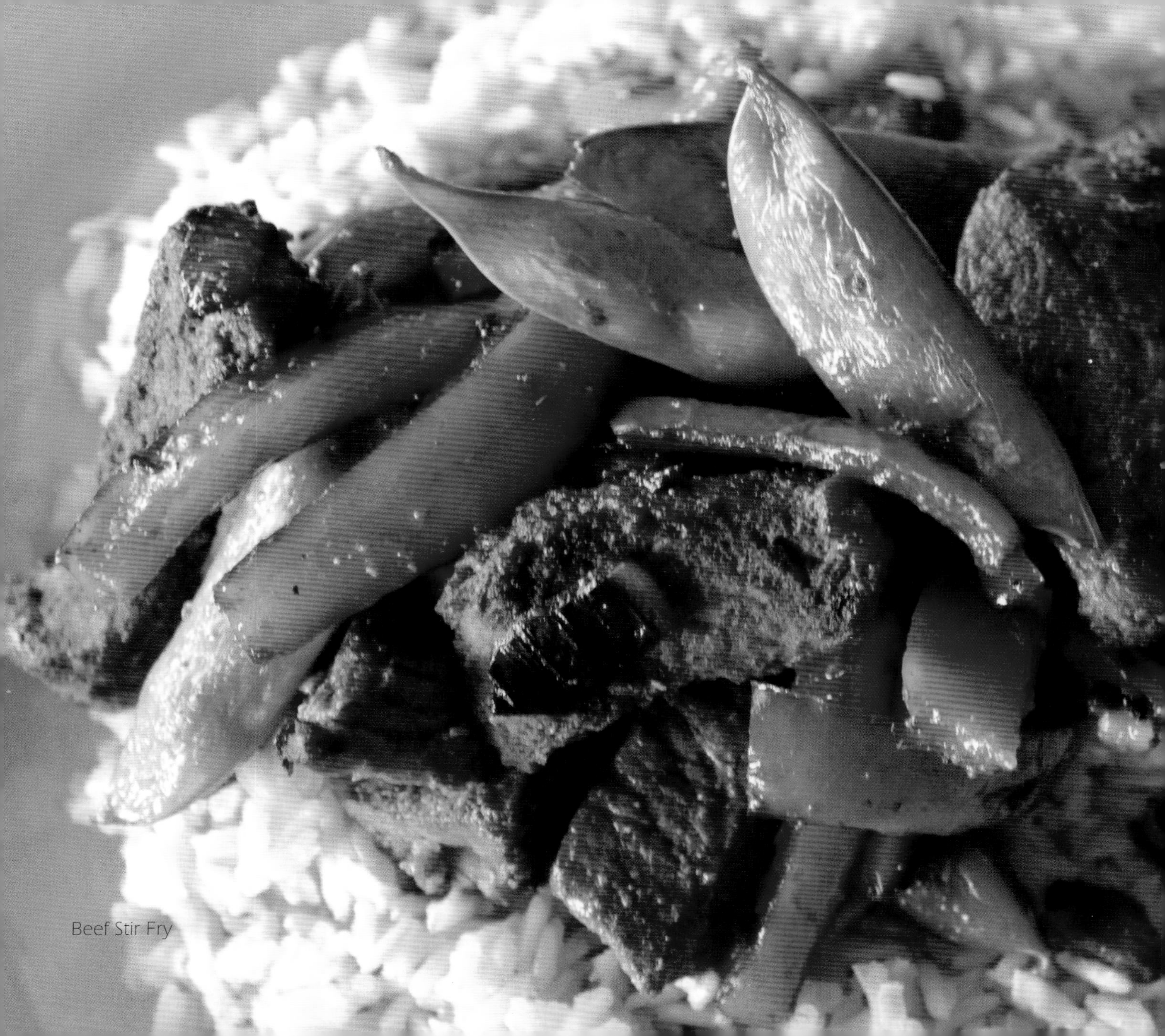

Beef Stir Fry

Steak with Jicama Salsa

- ½ tsp. cumin
- ½ tsp. oregano
- dash of salt and pepper
- 4–8 oz. **beef sirloin/steak**

Salsa

- ¼ cup **mango**, peeled and sliced
- ¼ cup jicama, peeled and sliced
- ¼ cup bell pepper
- 2 Tbsp. lemon juice
- ¼ tsp. **lemon zest**
- 1 Tbsp. **fresh cilantro**, chopped
- 1/8 tsp. coriander
- dash of salt and ground pepper

1. In a small bowl, combine cumin, oregano, salt, and pepper. Rub steak with seasoning.
2. Heat grill to medium-high heat. Place steak on grill and cover. Cook each side for 2–5 minutes, depending on how you like your steak. (Use the thumb test on page 77 to determine tenderness.)
3. In a medium bowl, combine mango, jicama, bell pepper, lemon juice, lemon zest, cilantro, coriander, salt, and pepper. Transfer steak to a plate. Top with salsa.

Tacos with Mango Salsa

- 4–6 oz. **ground beef**
- ½ cup **cheddar cheese**, shredded
- 1 Tbsp. **fresh cilantro**, chopped
- 2 **corn tortillas**
- 2 Tbsp. **sour cream**

Salsa

- 1 Tbsp. vegetable oil
- 2 Tbsp. **red onions**, chopped
- ¼ cup **mango**, peeled and chopped
- ¼ cup **pineapple** (canned, with juice)
- 2 Tbsp. honey
- 1 Tbsp. **lime juice**
- 2 tsp. white wine vinegar
- ¼ tsp. cornstarch

1. Sauté ground beef for 5–7 minutes over medium heat, until browned.
2. In a sauce pot over medium-high heat, add vegetable oil and onions and cook for 4 minutes. Add mango, pineapple, honey, lime juice, and vinegar. Bring to a boil. Turn down heat to a simmer and cook for 5 minutes. Add cornstarch to thicken salsa.
3. Divide beef, cheese, and mango salsa evenly and fill each tortilla. Garnish with sour cream and cilantro.

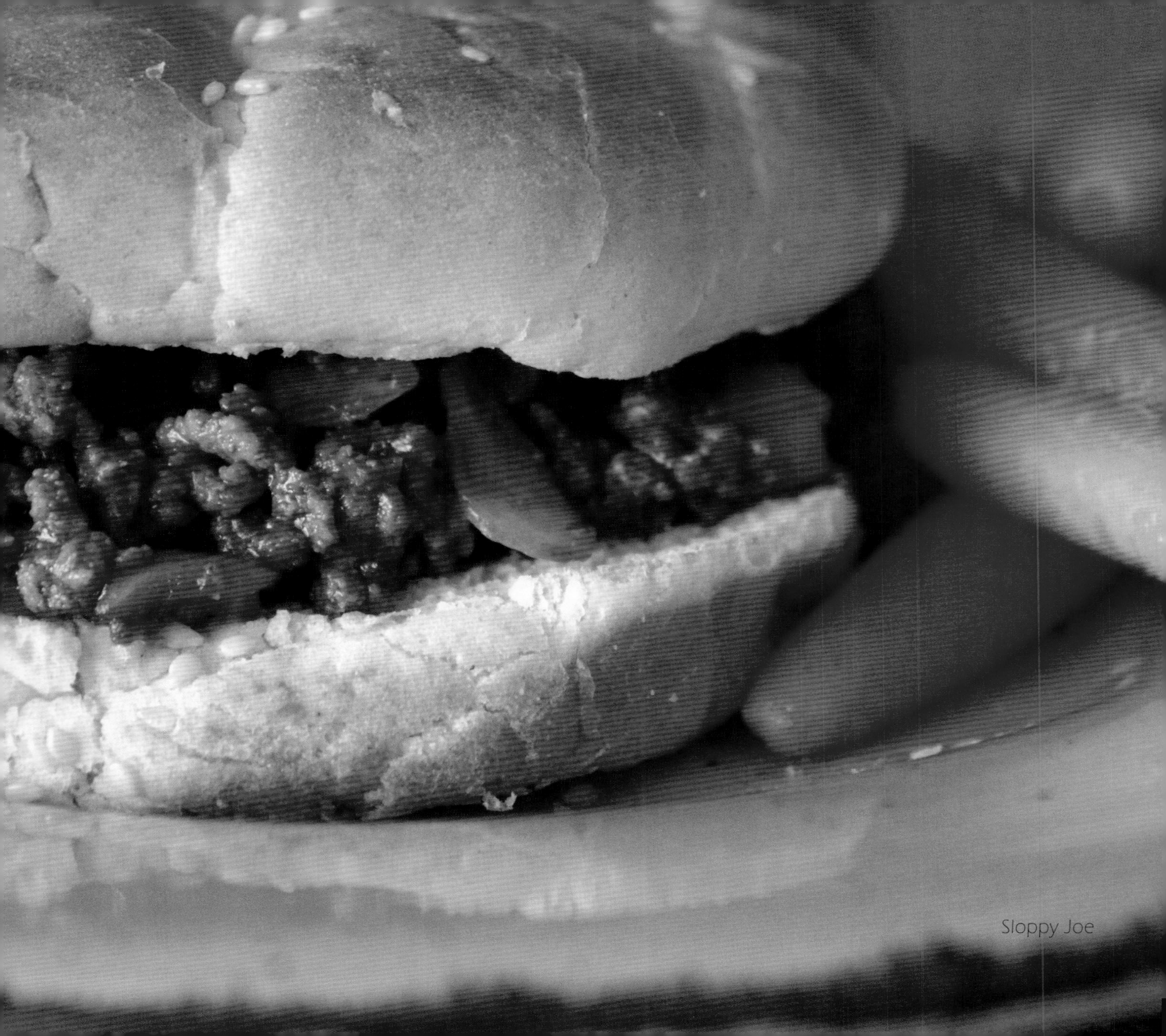

Sloppy Joe

Sloppy Joe

- 4–6 oz. **ground beef**
- 2 Tbsp. **yellow onion**, chopped
- ¼ tsp. garlic powder
- ¼ tsp. **stone-ground mustard**
- 2 Tbsp. **ketchup**
- ½ tsp. brown sugar
- dash of salt and pepper
- 1 **hamburger bun**

1. Cook ground beef in a medium skillet for 5–7 minutes over medium-high heat, until browned. Add onions and cook for another 3 minutes.
2. Add garlic powder, mustard, ketchup, brown sugar, salt, and pepper. Mix well and let simmer for 1–2 minutes.
3. Dish meat mixture onto bun.

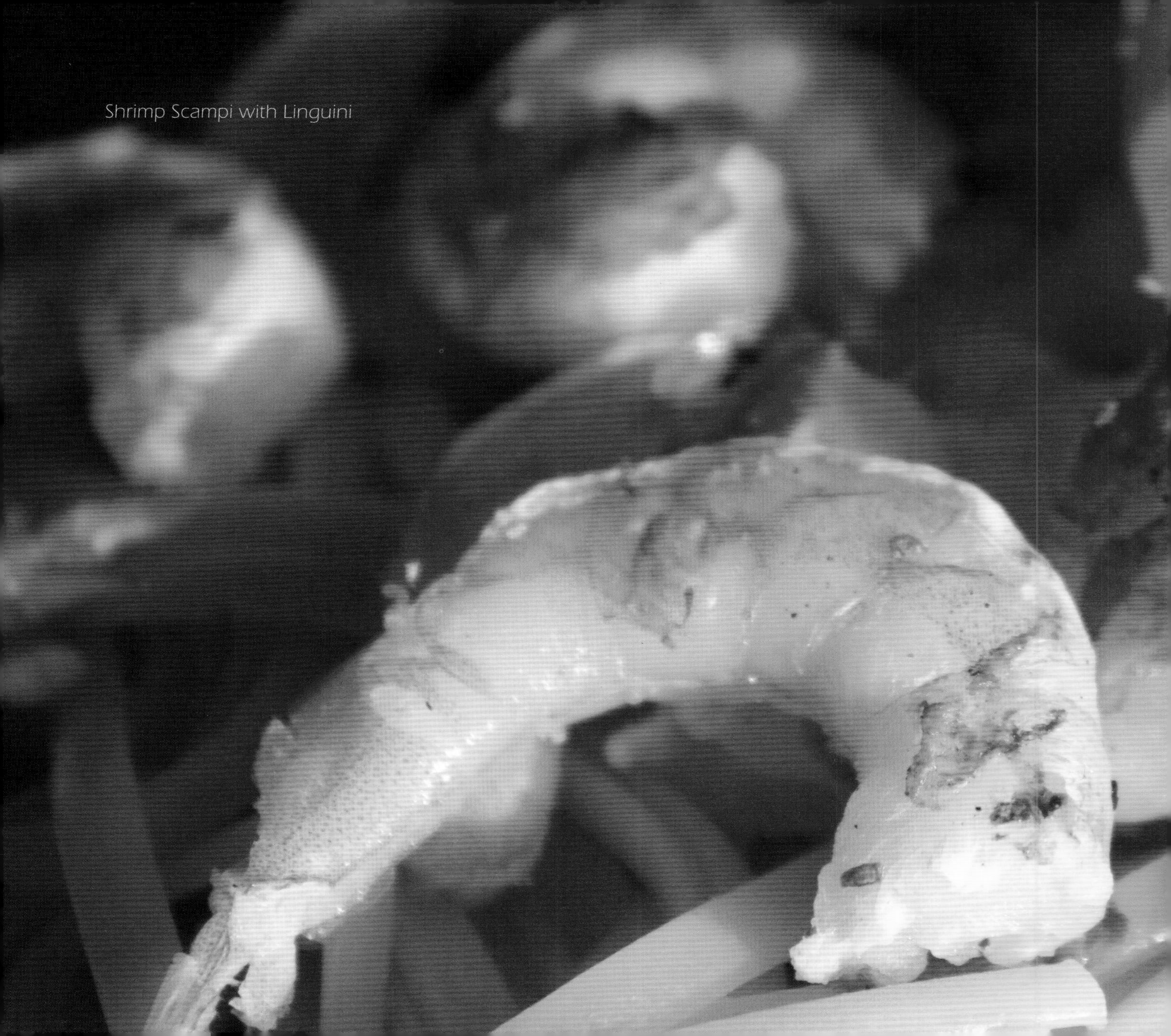

Shrimp Scampi with Linguini

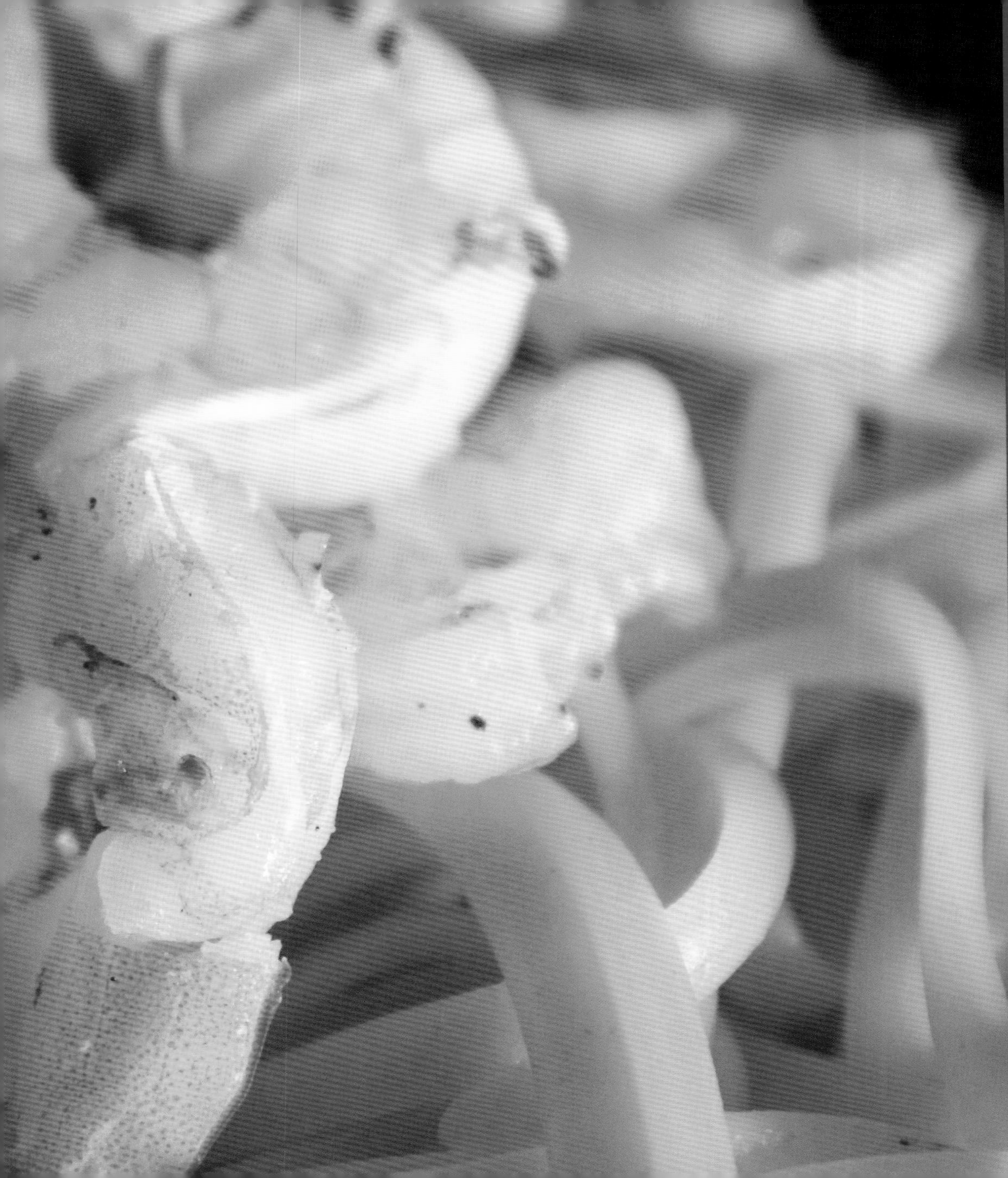

Seafood

Seafood

Cooking fish has always been an interesting adventure for me. I used to want to cook fish, but I didn't grow up eating more than fish sticks, so it always seemed so intimidating to me. My attempts on my own resulted in just trying to conquer the actual cooking of fish, rather than knowing how to season and dress it up. However, over the years, I have discovered the basics of preparing and cooking fish and other types of seafood. And because of that, I can officially say that anyone can do it.

Nutrition Facts

I'm sure you've heard that fish is good for you. It's true. Typically people on diets are counseled to eat fish in place of other meats. Let's take a look at some of the basic nutrition facts:[1]

Fish (3 oz cooked)	Calories (kcal)	Protein (g)	Total Fat (g)	Sat. Fat (g)
Cod	90	20	1	0
Halibut	120	23	2	0
Salmon	200	24	10	2
Shrimp	100	21	1.5	0
Tilapia	110	22	4	2.5
Trout (Rainbow)	140	20	6	2

1 U.S. Food and Drug Administration, www.fda.gov, (accessed 2/10/10).

Buying Seafood

I like to purchase my seafood from the butcher. That way I get the exact amount I want, and it is usually fresher. When buying shrimp, you can ask for the things you want such as deveined, peeled, and no tail.

Basic Types of Fish

It is good to review the basic types of fish and where they come from. There are three types of fish: saltwater, migratory, and freshwater.

Saltwater Fish

- Tilapia
- Trout

Migratory Fish

- Salmon

Freshwater Fish

- Cod
- Halibut

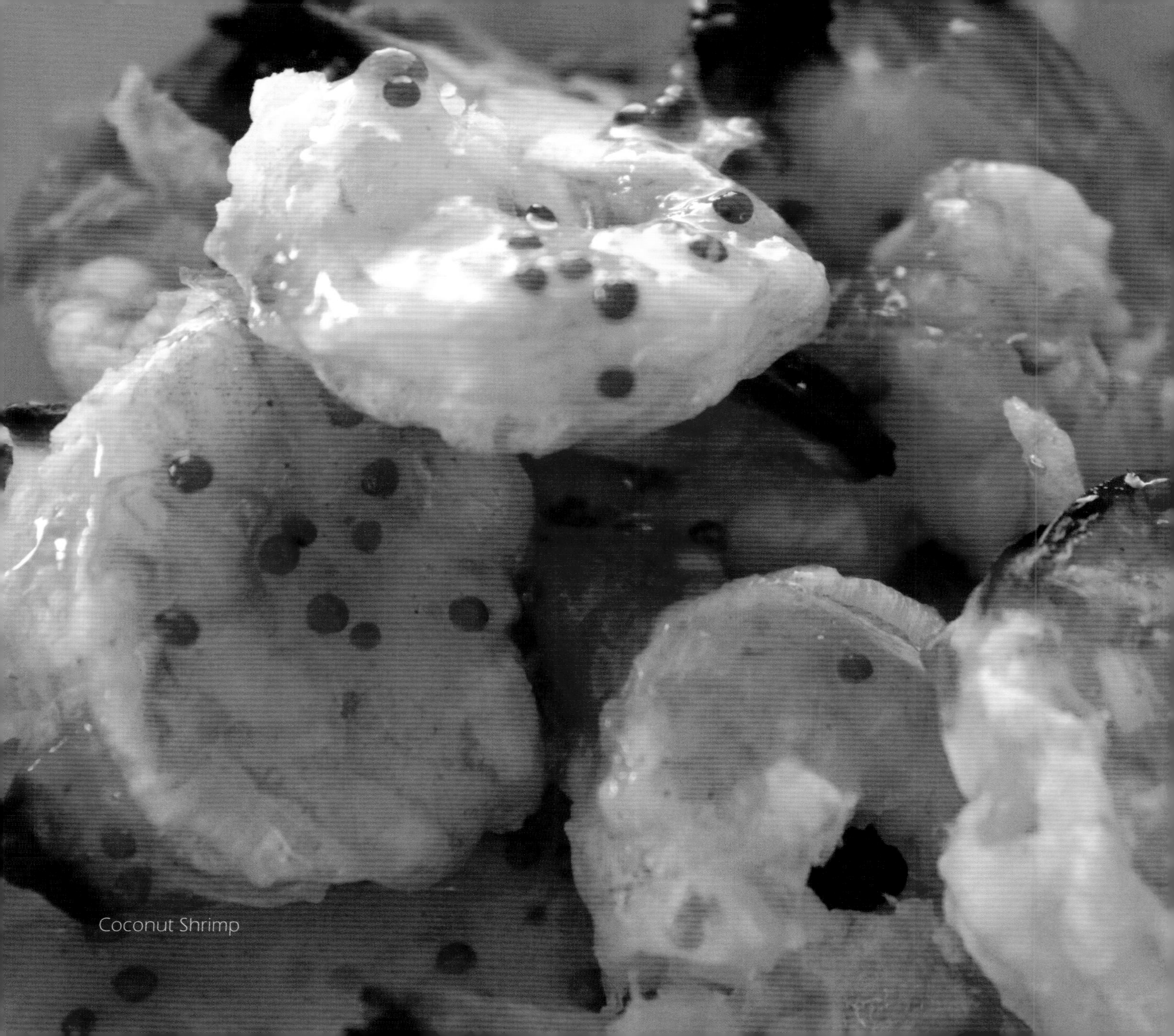

Coconut Shrimp

Coconut Shrimp

- 2 Tbsp. flour
- 2 Tbsp. white wine vinegar
- ¼ cup grated coconut, fresh if possible
- pinch of salt and pepper
- 4–6 oz. **shrimp**, peeled and deveined
- 2 Tbsp. mango or peach preserves
- 1 tsp. **stone-ground mustard**
- 1 Tbsp. **orange juice**

1. In a small bowl, combine flour, vinegar, coconut, salt, and pepper. Add shrimp and fully coat.
2. Heat broiler. Place shrimp on a greased baking sheet (drizzle the extra mix over the shrimp) and place in oven about 3–4 inches from the top. Broil for about 4 minutes on each side, until shrimp is opaque throughout.
3. Meanwhile, in a small saucepan, combine preserves, mustard, and orange juice. Bring to a boil, stirring constantly. Let simmer for 5 minutes. Remove from heat.
4. Transfer shrimp to plate and drizzle glaze over the top.

Citrus Glazed Halibut

- 1 **halibut fillet**, 4–6 oz.
- 1 tsp. olive oil
- dash of salt and ground pepper
- 1 Tbsp. **orange juice**
- 1 tsp. lemon juice
- 1 tsp. brown sugar
- 1 Tbsp. honey
- dash of cloves
- ¼ cup grapefruit, chopped
- 1 tsp. **fresh cilantro**, chopped

1. Heat grill to medium-high heat. Rub fish with olive oil, salt, and pepper. Place halibut, skinned side up, on grill. Cover grill and cook each side for 5 minutes, or until opaque throughout.
2. Meanwhile, in a small saucepan, mix together orange juice, lemon juice, brown sugar, honey, and cloves. Bring mixture to a boil, stirring constantly. Let simmer for 5 minutes. Remove from heat.
3. Transfer halibut to a plate and drizzle citrus glaze on top. Garnish with grapefruit and cilantro.

Glazed Salmon

- 2 Tbsp. unsalted butter, melted
- 2 Tbsp. brown sugar
- 1 **salmon fillet**, 4–6 oz.

1. Preheat oven to 450 degrees. In a small bowl, combine butter and brown sugar. Coat salmon thoroughly.
2. Place salmon in a greased baking pan. Cover pan with aluminum foil and bake for about 30 minutes, until fish is opaque throughout. Transfer to a plate.

Pine-Apple Tilapia

- 1 **tilapia fillet**, 4–6 oz.
- 3 Tbsp. olive oil
- 1 Tbsp. **pineapple juice**
- 1 Tbsp. **chopped gala** or **red delicious apple**
- 2 Tbsp. apple cider vinegar
- 1 Tbsp. honey
- 1 Tbsp. **lime juice**
- ¼ tsp. garam masala

1. Combine all of the ingredients in a Ziploc bag. Seal the bag and shake until the contents are mixed thoroughly. Marinate for 30 minutes.
2. Heat broiler. Place tilapia on a greased baking pan. Broil for 8–10 minutes, until fish is opaque.

Honey Ginger Halibut

- 1 tsp. garlic, minced
- 1 Tbsp. honey
- 1 Tbsp. soy sauce
- 1 Tbsp. balsamic vinegar
- ¼ tsp. **fresh ginger**, grated
- 1 ½ tsp. olive oil
- dash of salt and pepper
- 1 **halibut fillet**, 4–6 oz
- 1 tsp. **sesame seeds**
- 2–3 **fresh parsley** leaves

1. In a small bowl, combine garlic, honey, soy sauce, balsamic vinegar, ginger, and ½ tsp. olive oil. Season halibut with salt and pepper. Brush mixture on halibut, reserving excess.
2. In a small skillet, add 1 tsp. olive oil and halibut. Sauté over medium heat for 4 minutes on each side, or until opaque throughout.
3. Meanwhile, in a small saucepan add remaining mixture and bring to a boil. Let simmer for 5 minutes.
4. Transfer halibut to a plate and drizzle with remaining ginger glaze. Garnish with sesame seeds and parsley.

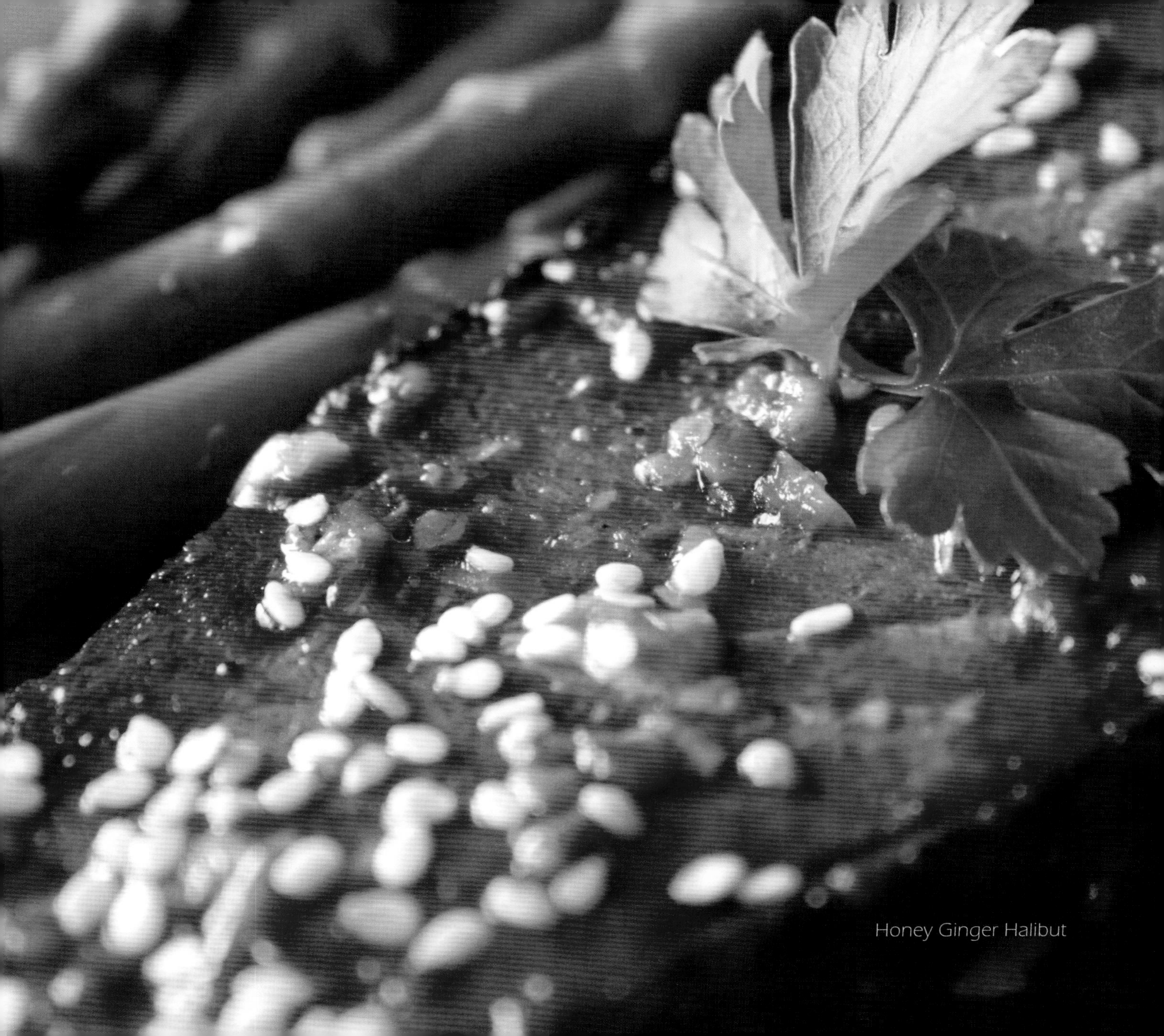

Honey Ginger Halibut

Lemon Trout with Tartar Sauce

- 1 Tbsp. butter, melted
- 3 tsp. lemon juice
- ¼ tsp. **lemon zest**
- 1 Tbsp. flour
- ¼ tsp. salt
- ¼ tsp. white pepper
- 1 **trout fillet**, 4–6 oz.

Tartar Sauce

- 2 Tbsp. **mayonnaise**
- 1½ tsp. sweet pickle relish
- 1 tsp. minced onion
- pinch of **fresh parsley**

1. Preheat oven to 350 degrees. In a small bowl, mix together butter, 2 tsp. lemon juice, and lemon zest. In another bowl mix together flour, salt, and white pepper. Dip trout into butter mixture and then in the flour mixture.
2. Place trout in a baking dish. Pour remaining butter mixture over the fish. Cook uncovered for 25–30 minutes, until fish flakes with fork.
3. Meanwhile, in another small serving bowl, add mayonnaise, relish, minced onion, remaining lemon juice, and parsley. Transfer fish to plate and serve with tartar sauce.

Mint Salmon

- 1 **salmon fillet**, 4–6 oz.
- ¼ tsp. coriander
- dash of salt and pepper
- 1 Tbsp. **fresh mint**, finely chopped
- 2 Tbsp. lemon juice
- 1 tsp. **fresh cilantro**, finely chopped
- 1 tsp. **green onion**, chopped
- ¼ tsp **fresh ginger**, minced
- 1 tsp. olive oil
- ½ cup **cantaloupe**, finely chopped

1. Season salmon with coriander, salt, and pepper. Heat grill to medium-high heat. Add salmon and cook for 3–5 minutes on each side, or until opaque throughout.
2. Meanwhile, in a small saucepan, mix together mint, lemon juice, cilantro, ginger, and olive oil. Bring to a boil. Add cantaloupe. Simmer for 5 minutes.
3. Transfer fish to a plate and drizzle mint mixture over the top.

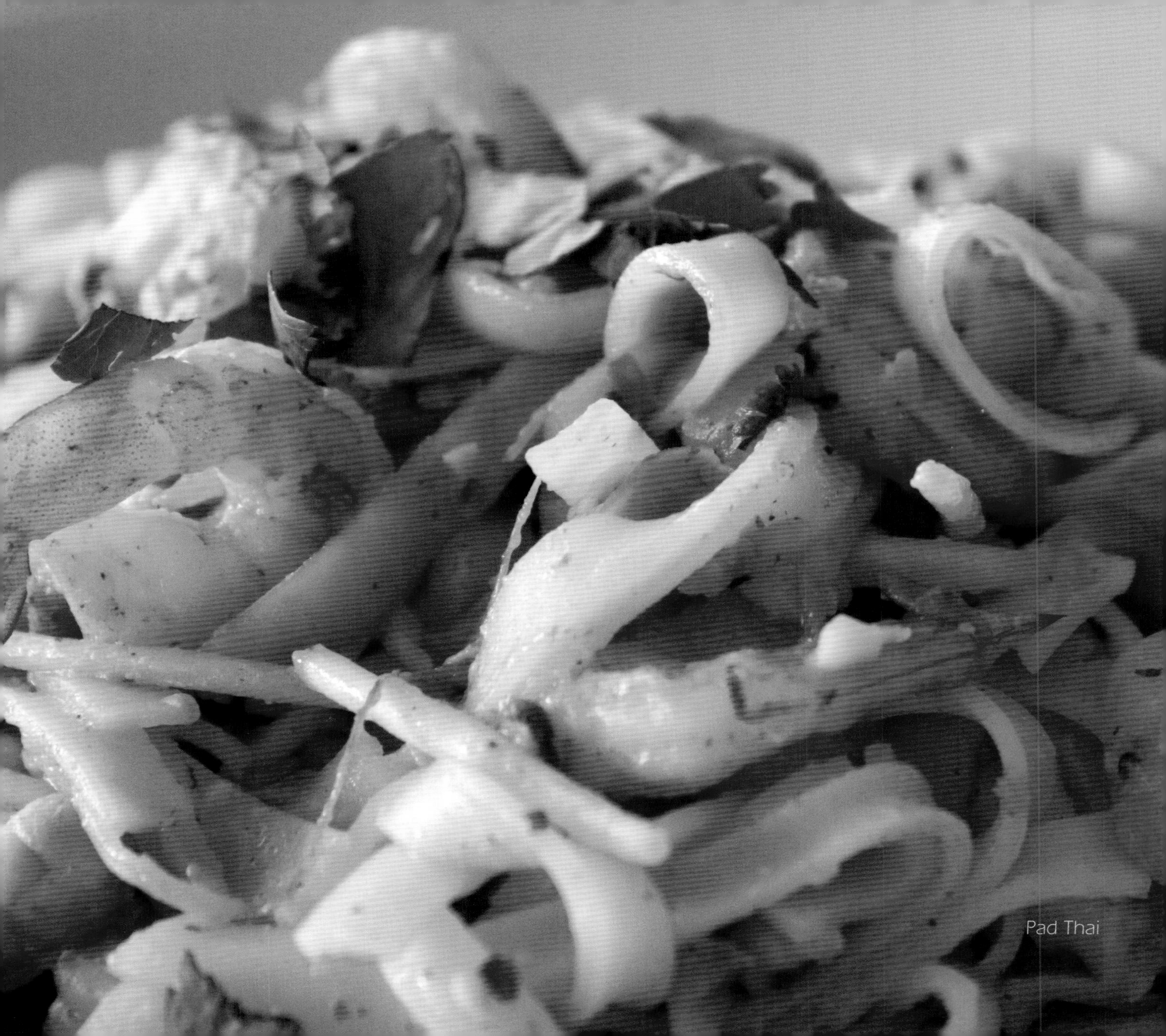

Pad Thai

Pad Thai

- 2–3 ounces rice noodles, linguini size
- 4–6 oz. **shrimp**, peeled, deveined, and with tails removed
- 1 Tbsp. fish sauce
- 1 tsp. rice vinegar
- 1 tsp. water
- 1 tsp. sugar
- 1½ tsp. Thai green chiles
- 3 tsp. garlic, minced
- 1 Tbsp. olive oil
- ½ cup **bean sprouts** (plus extra for garnish)
- ¼ cup **green onions**, julienne
- 1 tsp. egg, whisked
- 1 Tbsp. **fresh cilantro**, chopped
- 1 Tbsp. peanuts, dry-roasted

1. Fill a small saucepan with water and bring to a boil. Remove from heat and soak rice noodles for about 25 minutes, until softened. Drain and let cool.
2. In small bowl, combine fish sauce, rice vinegar, water, sugar, 1½ tsp. garlic, and Thai green chiles. Set aside.
3. In a medium skillet, heat remaining garlic, olive oil, and shrimp. Cook for 3–5 minutes, until shrimp is browned on both sides and opaque in the center.
4. Add noodles, fish sauce mixture, ½ cup bean sprouts, green onions, and egg. Mix until noodles are coated. Cook for about 3 minutes.
5. Transfer to plate and garnish with remaining bean sprouts, cilantro, and peanuts.

Rosemary Salmon

- 3 Tbsp. olive oil
- ½ tsp. garlic, minced
- 1 tsp. red wine vinegar
- 1 ½ tsp. lemon juice
- ½ tsp. **lemon zest**
- 2 tsp. **fresh rosemary**, crushed
- 1 tsp. sugar
- ¼ tsp. oregano
- ¼ tsp. ground coriander
- pinch of salt and pepper
- 1 **salmon fillet**, 4–6 oz.

1. In a Ziploc bag, combine 2 Tbsp. olive oil, garlic, vinegar, lemon juice and zest, rosemary, sugar, oregano, coriander, salt, and pepper. Seal bag and shake until contents are mixed thoroughly.
2. Place salmon in Ziploc bag, coat thoroughly, and marinate for 30 minutes.
3. Heat grill to medium-high heat. Rub salmon with 1 Tbsp. olive oil, salt, and pepper. Place salmon on grill, skinned side up. Cover grill and cook each side for 4–5 minutes, or until opaque throughout.

Salmon with Kiwi Chutney

- 1 **salmon fillet**, 4–6 oz.
- ¼ tsp. ground coriander
- dash of salt and ground pepper
- 1 tsp. vegetable oil
- ¼ cup **red onion**, chopped
- ¼ tsp. garlic, minced
- ¼ tsp. **fresh ginger**, minced
- ½ tsp. **jalapeño pepper**, seeded and diced
- ¼ cup **fresh peach**, chopped
- 1½ tsp. brown sugar
- 1 Tbsp. white wine vinegar
- 1 kiwi, chopped
- 1 tsp. **fresh cilantro**, chopped

1. Season salmon with coriander, salt, and pepper. Heat grill to medium-high heat. Add seasoned salmon and cook for 4–5 minutes on each side, or until opaque throughout.
2. In a sauce pot over medium-high heat, add oil, onions, garlic, ginger, and jalapeño. Cook for 3–5 minutes, or until onion is tender. Add peach, brown sugar, vinegar, and 1 tsp. water. Bring to a boil. Turn down the heat to a simmer and cook 5 minutes. Remove from heat and mix in the kiwi.
3. Transfer salmon to a plate and top with chutney. Garnish with cilantro.

Pineapple Glazed Salmon

- ¼ cup **pineapple juice**
- ¼ cup **pineapple chunks**
- ¼ tsp. **fresh ginger**, grated
- 1 Tbsp. brown sugar
- 1 Tbsp. honey
- dash of cinnamon
- 1 **salmon fillet**, 4–6 oz.

1. Preheat oven to 450 degrees. In a small saucepan, whisk together pineapple juice and chunks, ginger, brown sugar, honey, and cinnamon. Bring mixture to a boil, stirring constantly. Reduce heat and simmer for 1–3 minutes, or until syrupy. Remove from heat.
2. In a small baking dish, add salmon and apply half of glaze over the top. Cover with aluminum foil and bake for 30–35 minutes, until fish is opaque throughout.
3. Transfer salmon to a plate and add remaining glaze to the finished meat.

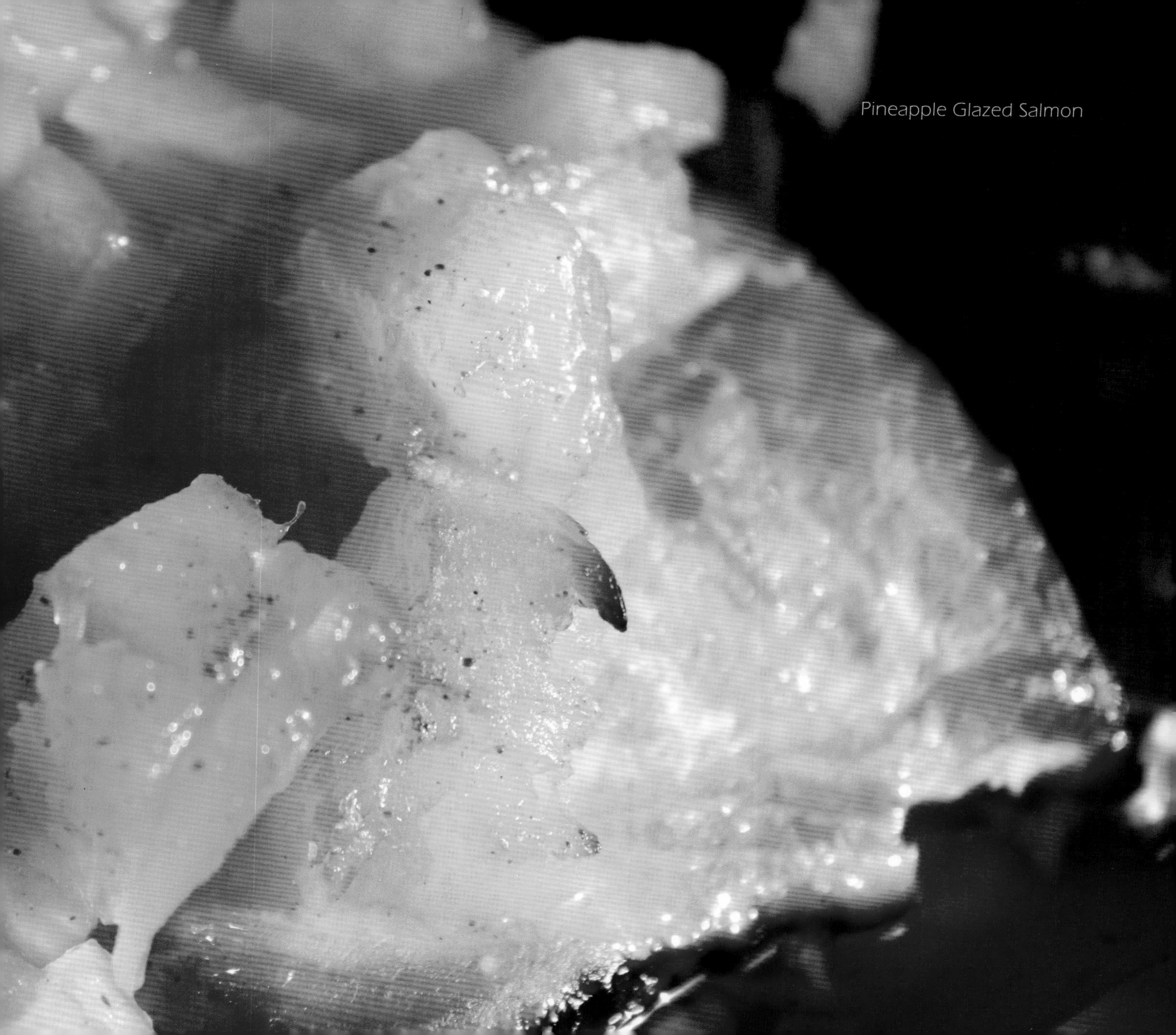

Pineapple Glazed Salmon

Shrimp Pasta

- 1½ Tbsp. olive oil
- 4–6 oz. **shrimp**, peeled, deveined, and tails removed
- dash of salt and pepper
- 1 tsp. garlic, minced
- ½ cup **stewed tomatoes**
- ½ cup water, plus extra for noodles
- ½ cup **grape tomatoes**
- 4–6 oz. angel hair pasta
- 1–2 Tbsp. **fresh basil**, chopped
- 1 tsp. **Parmesan cheese**, grated

1. In a small skillet, heat 1 Tbsp. olive oil. Season shrimp with salt and pepper and add to skillet. Sauté on medium heat for 3–5 minutes, until browned on both sides and opaque in the center.
2. In a small saucepan, add ½ Tbsp. olive oil, garlic, stewed tomatoes, and water. Bring to a boil. Reduce heat and let simmer for 15 minutes. Remove from heat and add grape tomatoes.
3. Meanwhile, fill a medium saucepan with water and bring to a boil. Add pasta and cook as instructed on the package. Drain and return to pan.
4. Add sauce and shrimp to pasta and mix well. Transfer to plate. Garnish with basil and Parmesan cheese.

Shrimp Scampi with Linguini

- 1 Tbsp. white wine (or white wine vinegar)
- 1 tsp. lemon juice
- 1 tsp. olive oil
- rosemary
- dash of salt and pepper
- 4–6 oz. **shrimp**, peeled, deveined, and tails removed
- 1 tsp. unsalted butter
- 1 tsp. garlic, minced
- 2–3 oz. linguini
- ¼ tsp. **lemon zest**
- 1 tsp. **fresh parsley**, chopped

1. In a Ziploc bag, add white wine, lemon juice, olive oil, rosemary, salt, and pepper. Mix well. Add shrimp and marinate for 30 minutes in the refrigerator.
2. Melt 1 tsp. butter in a small skillet. Add shrimp and garlic. Sauté for 5–7 minutes over medium heat, stirring occasionally, until shrimp is opaque in the center. Empty contents of Ziploc bag and bring to a boil. Reduce heat and simmer for 2–3 minutes, until marinade is mostly gone.
3. Meanwhile, fill a small saucepan with water and bring to a boil. Add pasta and cook as instructed on the package. Drain and return to pan.
4. Toss linguini with shrimp mixture. Transfer to a plate and garnish with lemon zest and parsley.

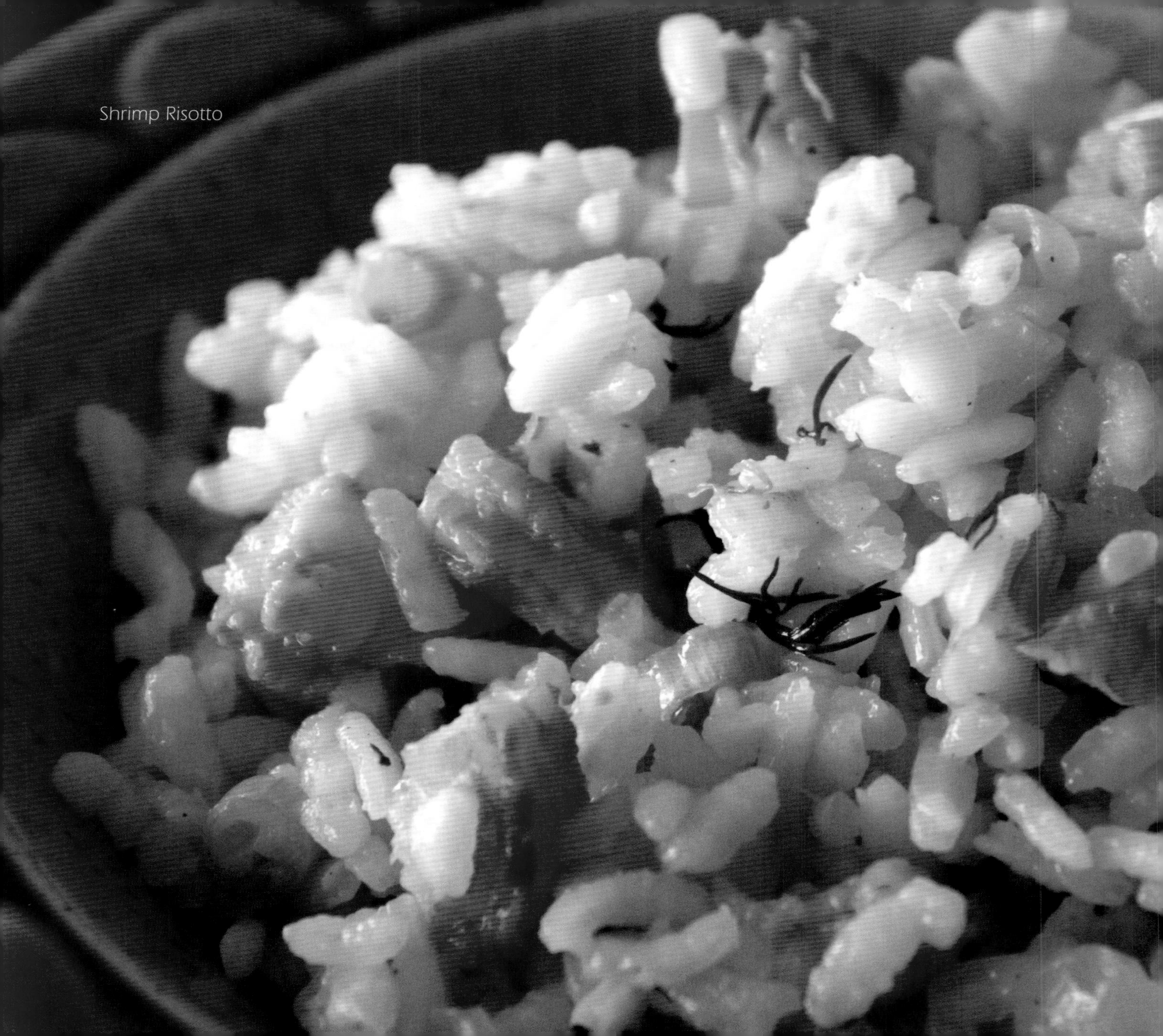
Shrimp Risotto

Shrimp Risotto

- 2 Tbsp. butter
- 1 Tbsp. **Worcestershire sauce**
- 1 tsp. garlic, minced
- ½ tsp. lemon pepper
- 3–4 oz. **shrimp**, peeled, deveined, and tails removed
- ¼ cup **yellow onions**, chopped
- ½ cup **Arborio rice**
- ¼ cup white wine (or white grape juice)
- 1 cup chicken broth
- ¼ cup **green onion**, chopped
- 1 tsp. dill weed
- ½ tsp. lemon juice
- ¼ tsp. **lemon zest**

1. In a small saucepan, melt 1 Tbsp. butter. Add Worcestershire sauce, garlic, and lemon pepper. Remove from heat and add shrimp. Coat fully.
2. In a small skillet, add shrimp and sauté over medium heat for 3–5 minutes, until opaque in the center. Cool and cut into small pieces.
3. Melt 1 Tbsp. butter in a medium saucepan. Add onions and sauté for 3–5 minutes over medium-low heat. Add rice and white wine. Stir and let cook for 2 minutes. Add half of the chicken broth. Cook for 7–10 minutes, until most of broth is absorbed. Repeat with rest of broth.
4. Add shrimp, green onions, dill, lemon juice, and lemon zest to risotto. Mix well.

Gnocchi with Tomato Sauce

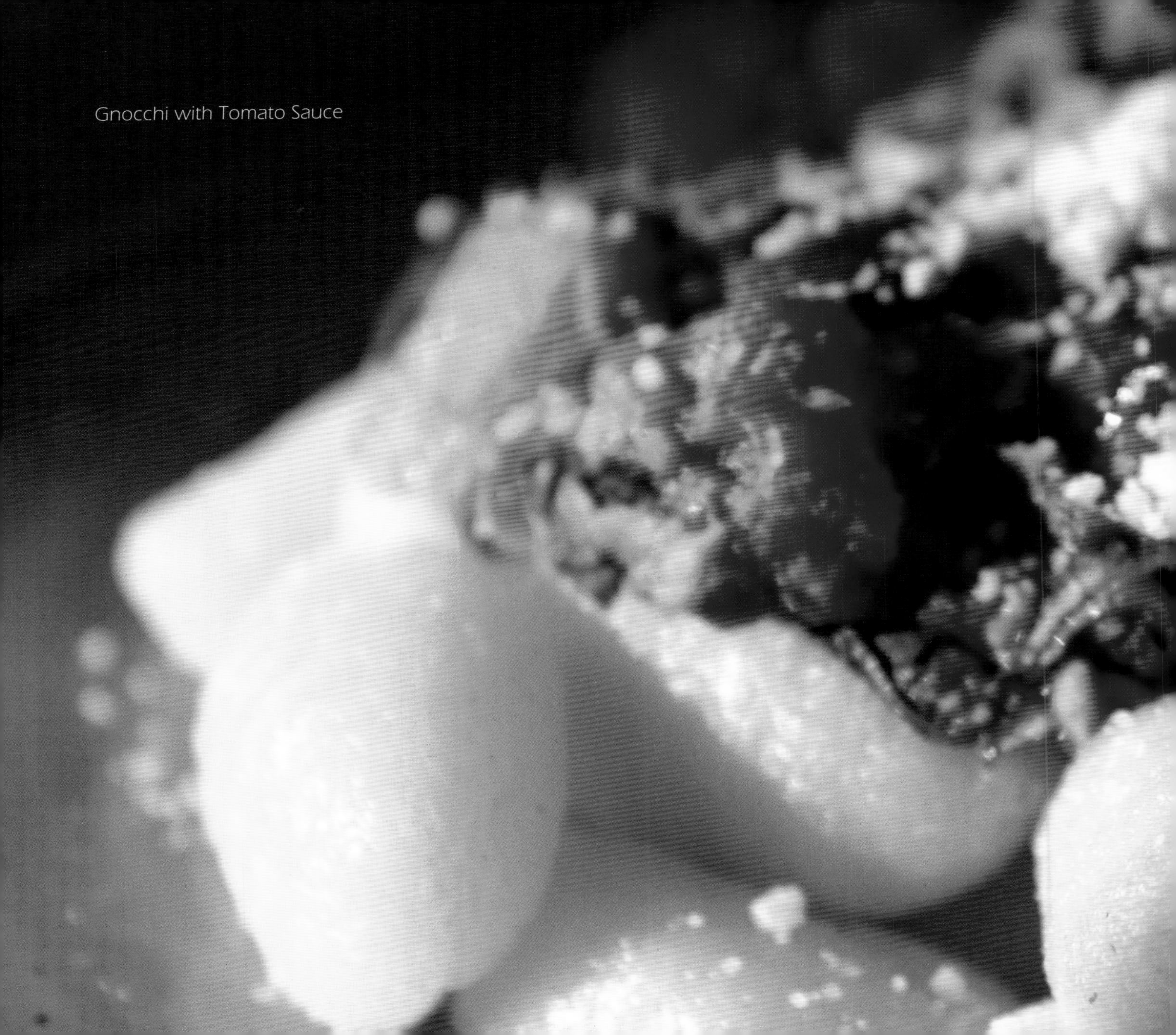

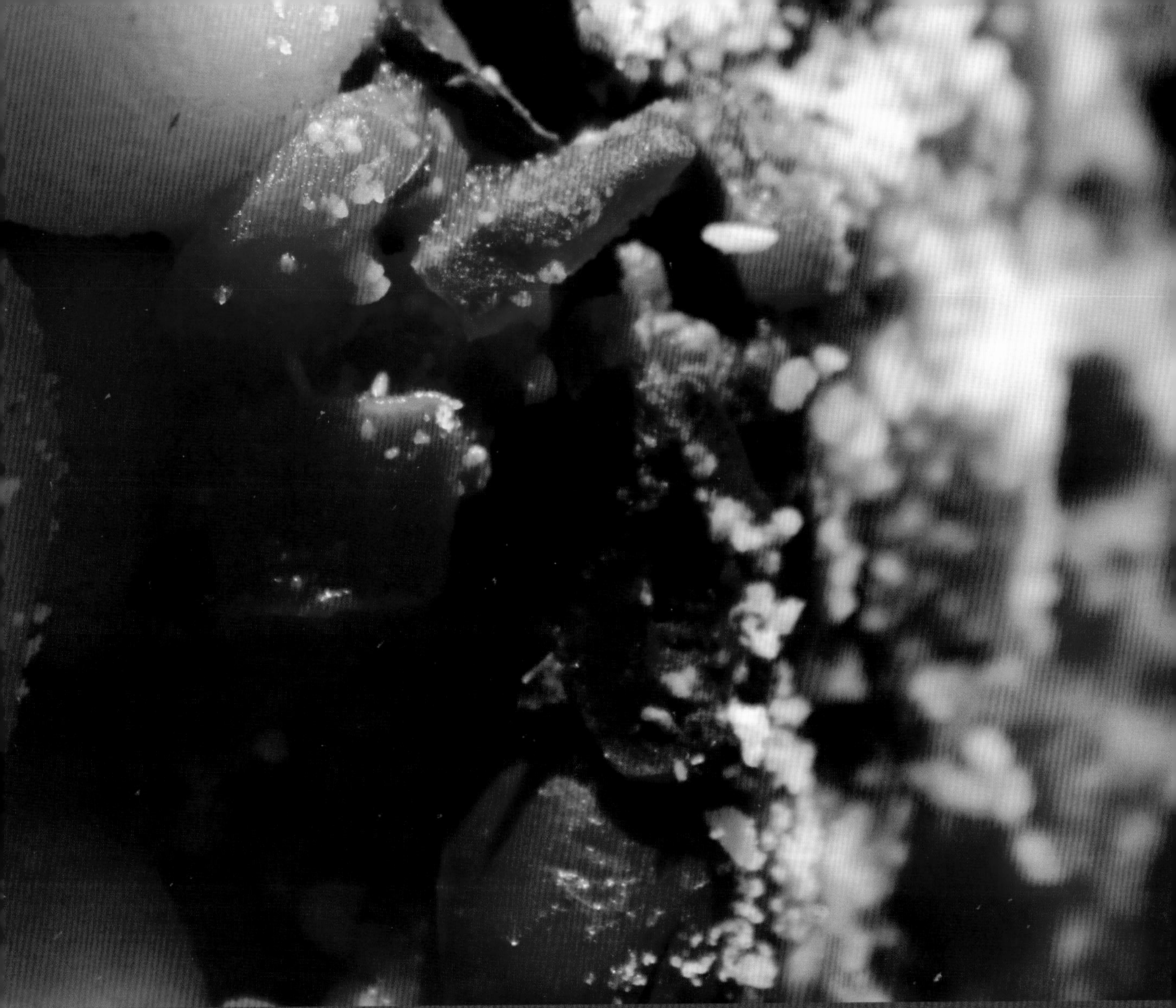

Grains

Grains

Grains encompass a variety of foods: pasta, rice, and breads. In other words, this section has it all. But each type of grain has a unique contributing ingredient, so let's learn a little bit more about each type of grain.

Rice

Rice is a staple food in most people's diets. While it often acts as a filler, it can also be the main dish. Rice can be used in a variety of ways. When I first started cooking, I considered it a small accomplishment to simply cook the rice, and usually forgot that I needed to add something to the rice or put something on top of it to make it a meal. Additionally, I would usually cook way too much rice for one and end up throwing away all of the leftovers. It has taken awhile to come up with ways to cook rice that will serve just one, but these recipes leave you with just the right amount.

Types of Rice

- **Short-grain rice**—This type of rice is round and fat. It is known to get sticky due to its high starch content.
- **Medium-grain rice**—This type of rice is sticky and has a tendency to clump together when it cools.
- **Long-grain rice**—This type of rice is long and has a low starch content, which is the reason it is often fluffy and dry.

Pasta

Pasta is also a staple in many diets, and there are a variety of types to choose from. I have specified specific types of pasta in the following recipes, but you are welcome to interchange pastas. Let's take a look at the basic types of pasta.[1]

- **Angel Hair**—The thinnest of all pasta. It is a long, fine, delicate, round strand.
- **Conchiglie (shells)**—A shell-type pasta that comes in regular and large sizes.
- **Couscous**—Round granules of pasta; one of the smallest types of pasta.
- **Egg Noodles**—Slightly twisted noodles. The egg provides richer flavor and color.
- **Elbow Macaroni**—A short, curved, semicircular tube.
- **Farfalle (bowtie)**—A pasta that looks like a bowtie or butterfly.
- **Fettuccine**—A ribbon-shaped strand; one of the most popular pastas.
- **Fusilli (twists)**—Fusilli means "little spindles," and looks like a corkscrew or twist.
- **Gnocchi**—Gnocchi is Italian for "dumpling"; it is usually filled with a type of potato.
- **Linguini**—A narrow, flat version of round spaghetti, and a narrower version of fettuccine.
- **Manicotti—**A stuffed, baked pasta, about 4 inches long.
- **Pastina**—Tiny little stars, one of the smallest types of pasta.
- **Penne**—Penne is Italian for "quills." It is a large, straight tube, cut diagonally.
- **Ravioli**—Stuffed pasta shaped like a pillow (circle or square).
- **Rigatoni**—A large, ribbed, slightly curved pasta, in the shape of a tube.
- **Ruote (wheel)**—Pasta shaped like a wheel with spokes.
- **Spaghetti**—The most famous cut of pasta. A long, round, thin, cordlike shape.
- **Tortellini**—A small, stuffed, twisted triangle-shaped pasta.
- **Ziti**—A medium-sized, long, thin, tubular-shaped pasta.

---

1 Referenced www.thenibble.com.

Butternut Squash Risotto

- 2 Tbsp. butter
- ½ cup **butternut squash**, peeled and chopped
- ¼ cup **yellow onion**, chopped
- 1 tsp. garlic, minced
- ¼ tsp. kosher salt
- ½ cup **Arborio rice**
- ¼ cup white wine (or white grape juice)
- 1 cup chicken broth
- ¼ cup gouda cheese
- 1 tsp. **fresh sage**, chopped
- pinch of ground pepper

1. Melt 1 Tbsp. butter in a small saucepan and add squash, onion, garlic, and salt. Sauté for about 15 minutes on medium-low heat, stirring occasionally, until butternut squash is tender. Remove from heat and set aside.
2. In another small saucepan, melt 1 Tbsp. butter and add rice and wine. Mix thoroughly. Let simmer until wine has almost evaporated. Add half the broth and cook for 8–10 minutes, until broth is almost absorbed. Repeat with the rest of the broth, stirring occasionally.
3. Add gouda and stir until cheese melts and risotto thickens. Season with salt, pepper, and sage.

Butternut Risotto

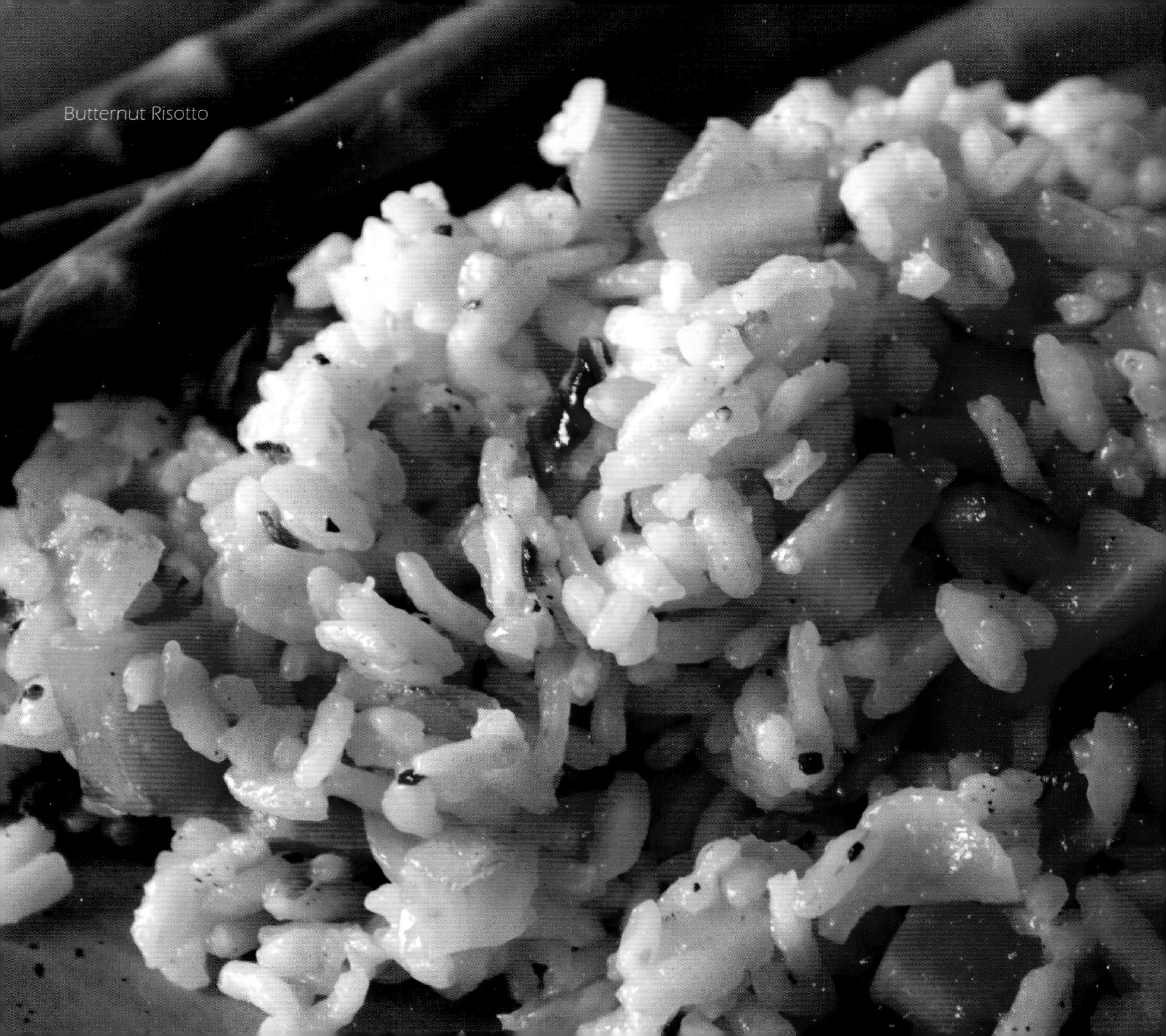

Gnocchi with Tomato Sauce

- 1½ cup gnocchi, uncooked
- 1 tsp. olive oil
- ¼ cup **yellow onions**, chopped
- 1 tsp. garlic, minced
- 1 cup **tomatoes**, chopped
- ¼ cup **stewed tomatoes**
- ¼ cup **fresh basil**, chopped
- 2 Tbsp. **kalamata olives**, sliced
- 1 tsp. **Parmesan cheese**, grated

1. Fill a medium saucepan with water and bring to a boil. Add gnocchi and cook as instructed on the package. Drain and return to pan.
2. Meanwhile, in a medium skillet add olive oil, onion, and garlic. Sauté for 3–5 minutes on medium heat until onion is tender. Add fresh tomatoes and cook 35 minutes, until tender. Add stewed tomatoes and simmer on medium-low for 10 minutes.
3. Stir basil and olives into the sauce and cook for a minute more. Transfer pasta to a plate and pour sauce over the top. Sprinkle with Parmesan cheese.

Fettuccine Alfredo

- 4–6 oz. **fettuccine**
- ½ cup **heavy whipping cream**
- 1 Tbsp. lemon juice
- 2 Tbsp. unsalted butter
- ¼ cup **Parmesan cheese**, grated
- ½ tsp. **lemon zest**
- pinch of nutmeg
- pinch of salt and white pepper

1. Fill a medium saucepan with water and bring to a boil. Add fettuccine and cook as instructed on the package. Drain and return to pan.
2. In a small saucepan, add cream, lemon juice, and butter. Cook for about 3 minutes, until butter melts. Remove from heat.
3. Mix sauce into pasta saucepan. Add Parmesan, lemon zest, nutmeg, salt, and white pepper. Place saucepan over low heat for about 2 minutes, until sauce thickens. Stir frequently.

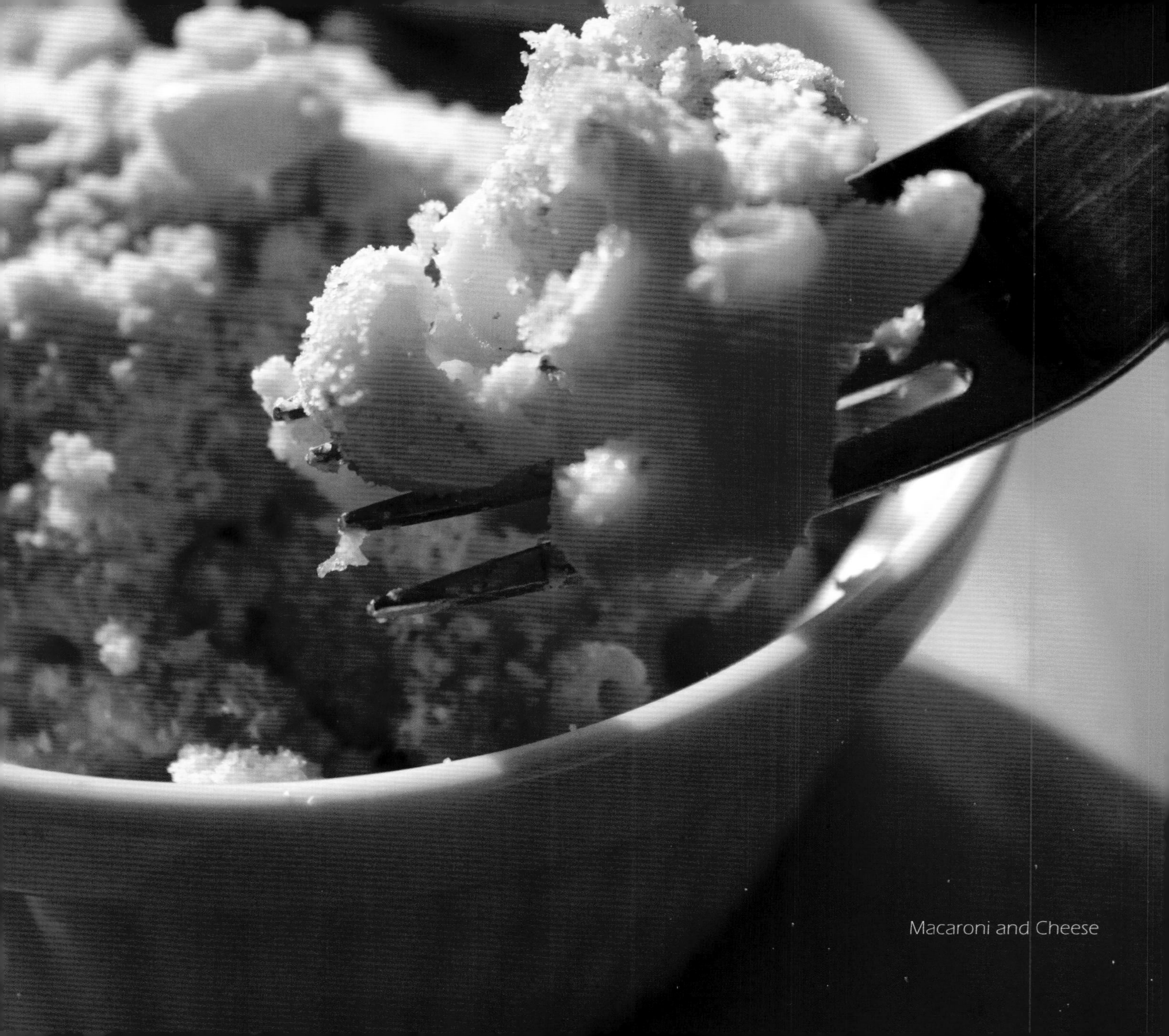

Macaroni and Cheese

Macaroni and Cheese

- 1 cup elbow pasta
- 2 Tbsp. butter
- 1 ½ tsp. flour
- ¼ cup milk
- ¼ cup **heavy whipping cream**
- dash of salt and ground pepper
- 1 cup **cheddar cheese**, shredded
- 2 tsp. **Parmesan cheese**, grated
- 1 Tbsp. **bread crumbs**

1. Preheat oven to 375 degrees. Fill small saucepan with water and bring to a boil. Add pasta and cook as instructed on the package. Drain and return to pan.
2. Meanwhile, in another small saucepan, melt 1 Tbsp. butter. Add flour, milk, cream, salt, and pepper. Bring to a boil. Reduce heat, add cheese, and stir until cheese is melted. Remove from heat and add pasta. Mix well. Transfer mixture to a 5-inch ramekin or baking dish.
3. Melt 1 Tbsp. butter in a small bowl. Drizzle butter over noodles. Sprinkle Parmesan cheese and bread crumbs over the top of noddle mixture. If using a ramekin, set it on a cookie sheet. Bake for 25 minutes. Remove from oven and let cool for 5 minutes.

Angel Hair with Basil Pesto

- 4–6 oz. angel hair pasta
- ½ cup **fresh basil**, chopped
- 1 ½ Tbsp. **Romano cheese**
- 1 Tbsp. olive oil
- 1 ½ tsp. **pine nuts**
- 1 tsp. garlic, minced
- pinch of salt and pepper

1. Fill a medium saucepan with water and bring to a boil. Add pasta and cook as instructed on the package. Drain and return to pan.
2. Combine basil, cheese, olive oil, pine nuts, garlic, salt, and pepper in a food processor or blender. Mix well until ingredients become a pasty sauce. Pour onto pasta and mix well.

Margarita Pizza

Dough

- ¼ cup warm water
- 1½ tsp. yeast
- 2½ tsp. sugar
- ¾ cup flour (preferably whole wheat)
- 2 tsp. extra virgin olive oil
- ½ tsp. salt
- 1 tsp. cornmeal

Toppings

- 1 tsp. olive oil
- 4–6 slices **mozzarella cheese**, sliced in rounds
- 4–6 slices **tomatoes**, round slices
- 3–4 fresh **basil leaves**, torn

1. Preheat oven to 375 degrees. In a small bowl combine water, yeast, and 1 tsp. sugar. Mix well. Add the rest of the sugar, flour, 1½ tsp. olive oil, and salt. Add more flour if needed.
2. Place dough on a floured surface. Knead until smooth. Let stand for 10 minutes. With a rolling pin, roll dough to desired shape. Spread ½ tsp. olive oil and cornmeal on a baking sheet. Place dough on top, and turn over to coat all of dough.
3. Brush dough with olive oil. Top with mozzarella rounds (enough to cover pizza) and tomatoes (enough to cover the pizza). Bake for 25 minutes. Let cool for 5 minutes. Garnish with fresh basil leaves.

Mushroom Fettuccine

- 4–6 oz. **fettuccine**
- 1 Tbsp. unsalted butter
- 1 Tbsp. flour
- ½ cup milk
- 1 Tbsp. **heavy whipping cream**
- pinch of salt and pepper
- 1 Tbsp. **Dijon mustard**
- 2 Tbsp. butter
- 1 tsp. garlic, minced
- 1 tsp. fresh thyme, chopped
- 1 cup **mushrooms**, sliced
- 3–4 **asparagus** stems

1. Fill a medium saucepan with water. Bring to a boil. Add fettuccine and cook as instructed on the package. Drain and return to pan.
2. Melt 1 Tbsp. butter in a small saucepan. Add flour, milk, cream, salt, and pepper. Bring to a boil. Stir for about 3 minutes, until mixture thickens. Remove from heat and stir in mustard.
3. Heat 1 Tbsp. butter in a medium skillet. Add garlic, thyme, mushrooms, and asparagus. Sauté for 10–15 minutes over medium heat until vegetables are tender. Toss together with pasta and sauce.

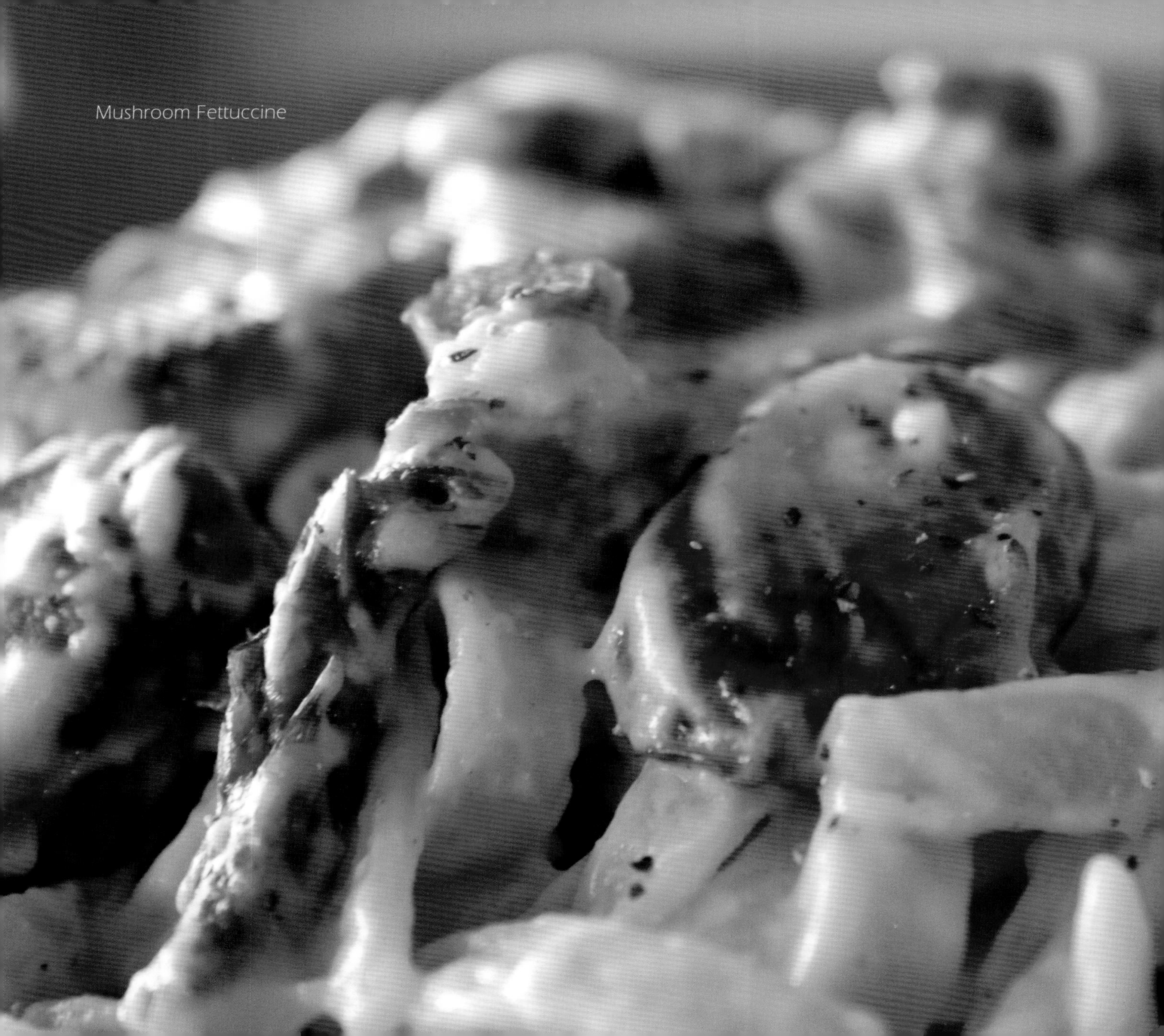

Mushroom Fettuccine

Mint Pesto Penne

- 1 cup penne pasta, uncooked
- ½ cup **fresh basil**, chopped
- ¼ cup **fresh mint**, chopped
- 1½ Tbsp. **Romano cheese**
- 1 Tbsp. olive oil
- 1½ tsp. **pine nuts**
- 1 tsp. garlic, minced
- ½ tsp. lemon juice
- pinch of salt and pepper

1. Fill a medium saucepan with water and bring to a boil. Add pasta and cook as instructed on the package. Drain and return to pan.
2. Combine basil, mint, cheese, olive oil, pine nuts, garlic, lemon juice, salt, and pepper in a food processor or blender. Mix well until it becomes a pasty sauce. Pour onto pasta and mix well.

Tomato-Pepper Pasta

- 4–6 oz. spaghetti
- 1 Tbsp. olive oil
- ¼ of a **green bell pepper**, julienne
- ¼ cup **yellow onion**, chopped
- 1 tsp. garlic, minced
- ½ cup **grape tomatoes**
- pinch of salt and pepper
- 1 tsp. **fresh basil**, chopped
- 1 Tbsp. **Parmesan cheese**, grated

1. Fill a medium saucepan with water and bring to a boil. Add spaghetti and cook as instructed on the package. Drain and return to pan.
2. In a small skillet over medium-low heat, sauté olive oil, green peppers, and onion for 3–5 minutes, or until the onions are tender. Stir occasionally.
3. Add garlic, tomatoes, salt, and pepper. Simmer for 5 minutes, or until tomatoes are soft, stirring occasionally. Remove from heat. Transfer pasta to a plate and top with green pepper and tomato mixture. Top with basil and cheese.

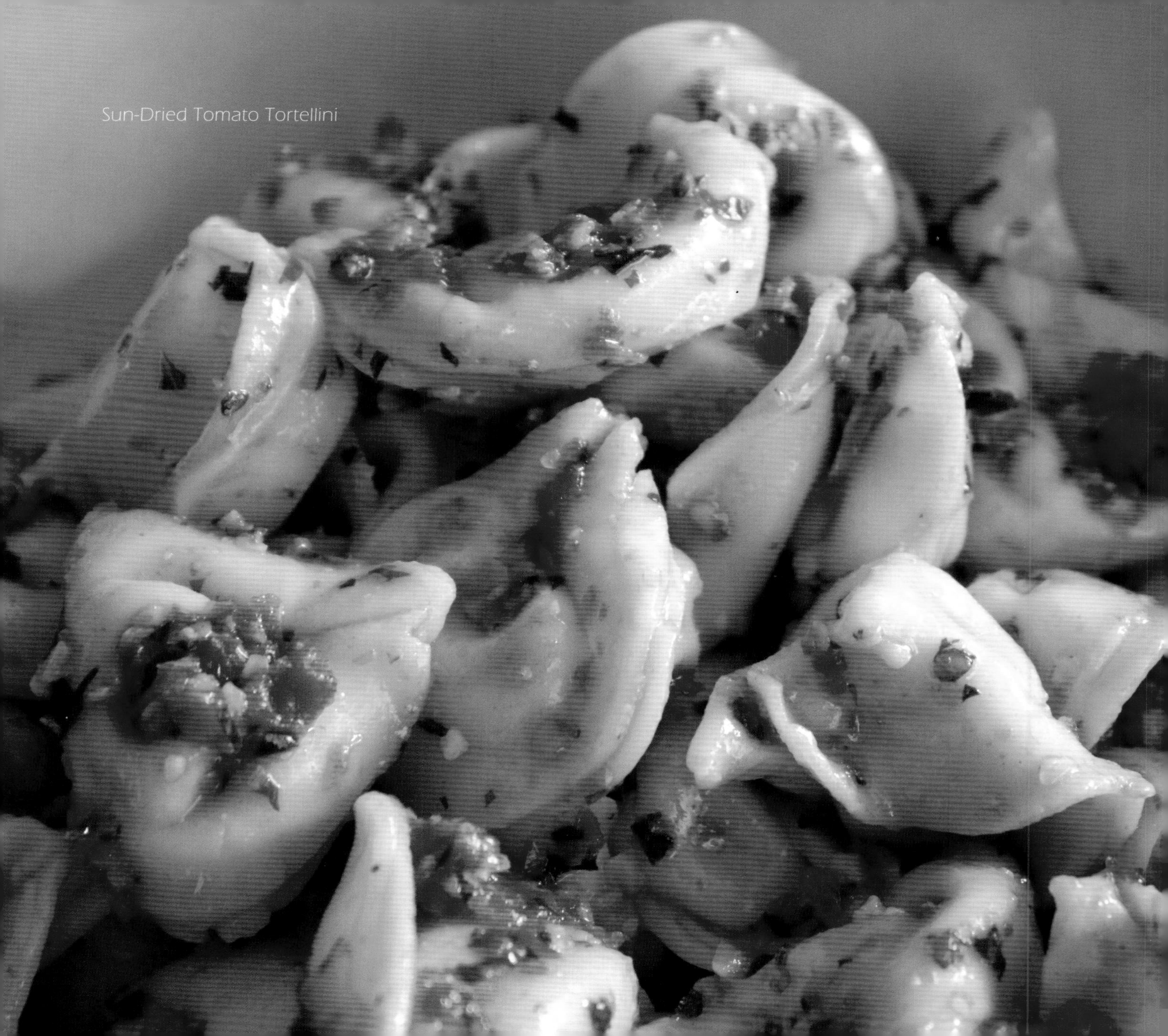

Sun-Dried Tomato Tortellini

Sun-Dried Tomato Tortellini

- 2 cups tortellini, uncooked
- ¼ cup **fresh basil**, chopped
- ¼ cup sun-dried tomatoes
- 1 ½ Tbsp. **Romano Cheese**
- 1 Tbsp. olive oil
- 1 Tbsp. **pine nuts**
- 1 tsp. garlic, minced
- ½ tsp. salt
- dash of pepper

1. Fill a medium saucepan with water and bring to a boil. Add tortellini and cook as instructed on the package. Drain and return to pan.
2. Combine basil, tomatoes, cheese, olive oil, pine nuts, garlic, salt, and pepper in a food processor or blender and mix until it becomes a pasty sauce. Pour mixture onto pasta and mix well.

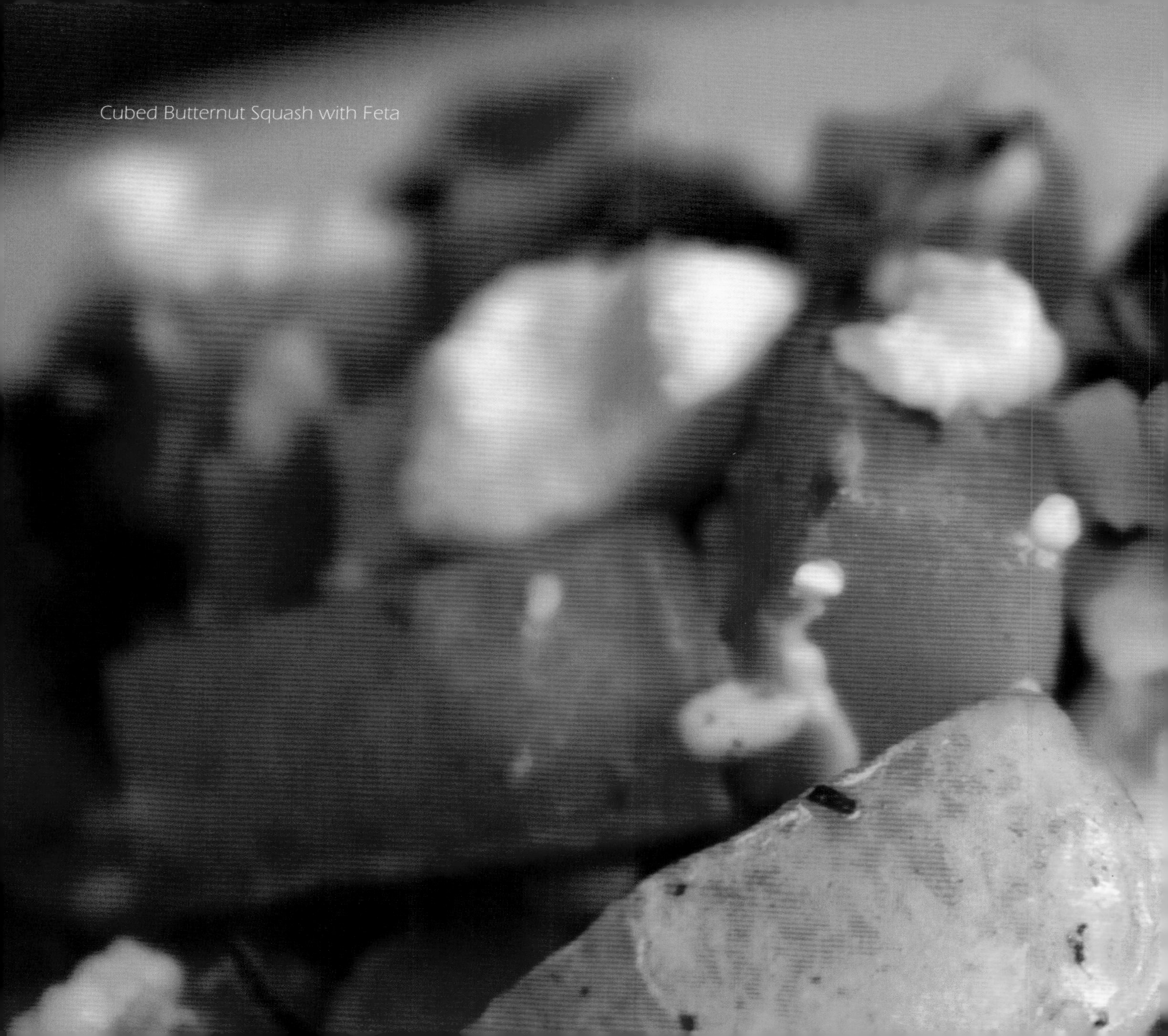
Cubed Butternut Squash with Feta

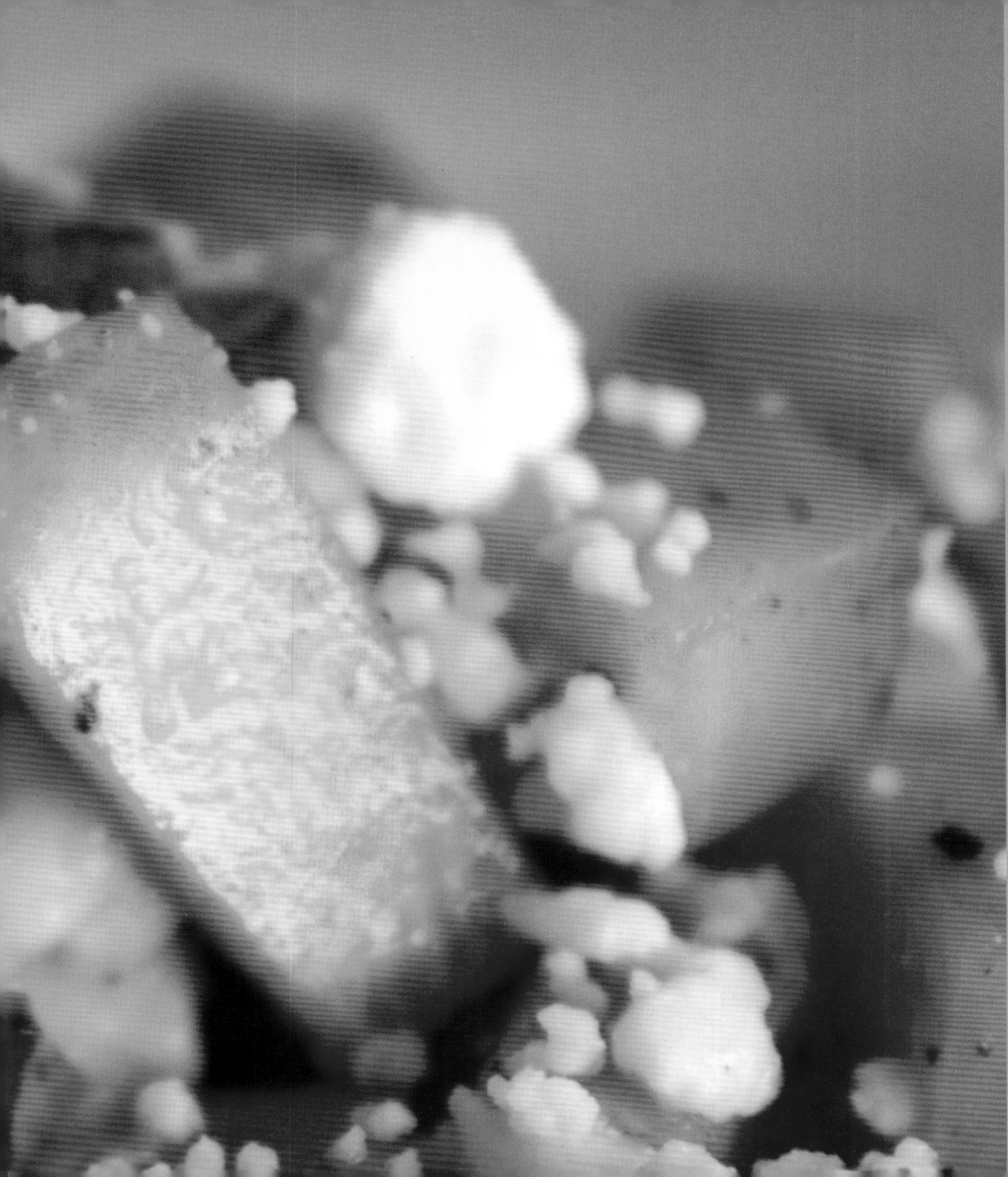

Side Dishes

Side Dishes

Side dishes can range from simple to extravagant. Usually side dishes are an afterthought, and as such, they run the risk of not complementing the meal. I have found that if I have both a sweet and savory option for my side dishes, I can make better pairings with my main dish. In this section I have included both sweet and sour options for you to choose from. But before we dive into recipes, I'd like to list some simple side dishes and cooking methods for you to consider.

Simple Side Dishes

These side dishes don't require a specific recipe. They are mostly just a vegetable or fruit chopped and served with a meal. After the list of simple side dishes are two cooking methods that can be applied to several of the vegetables.

Vegetables

- Green Beans (steamed or broiled)
- Broccoli (steamed or broiled)
- Green, Red, or Orange Bell Peppers (sliced julienne)
- Radishes (sliced or whole)
- Beets (sliced)
- Carrots (chopped, julienne, or whole; steamed, broiled, or fresh)
- Peas (steamed or boiled)

Fruit

- Apricot (dried or fresh, sliced)
- Banana (sliced)
- Blackberries
- Blueberries (better served with another berry)
- Cantaloupe (chopped)
- Cherries (on the stems or separated)
- Grapes (a handful on the vine or detached)
- Kiwi (sliced)
- Mango (dried or sliced)
- Oranges (peeled and sliced)
- Olives (assorted and sliced)
- Peach (sliced)
- Pineapple (chopped, and often soaked in honey)
- Plum
- Pear (sliced)
- Raspberries
- Strawberries (sliced or whole, sometimes with a dash of sugar)
- Watermelon (sliced or chopped)

Basic Vegetable Cooking Methods

Steaming

- **Stove Top**—Fill a pot until it just barely reaches the bottom of a colander or steamer basket. When the water comes to a boil, add the vegetables to the colander or steamer basket. Cover. Cook for 4–10 minutes, until vegetables are tender. Let cool.

- **Microwave**—Place vegetables in a microwave-safe bowl. Add water, fill to about half full. Cover with plastic wrap and poke one small hole in the top. Cook on high for 1–3 minutes, until vegetables are tender. Let cool.

Broiling

- Heat the broiler. Cut vegetables so that each are about the same thickness. Lay vegetables flat on a baking sheet, not overlapping. Drizzle olive oil and season with salt and pepper. Place baking sheet in the oven and cook for 1–5 minutes. Flip and cook for another 1–5 minutes, or until just browned and tender. Let cool.

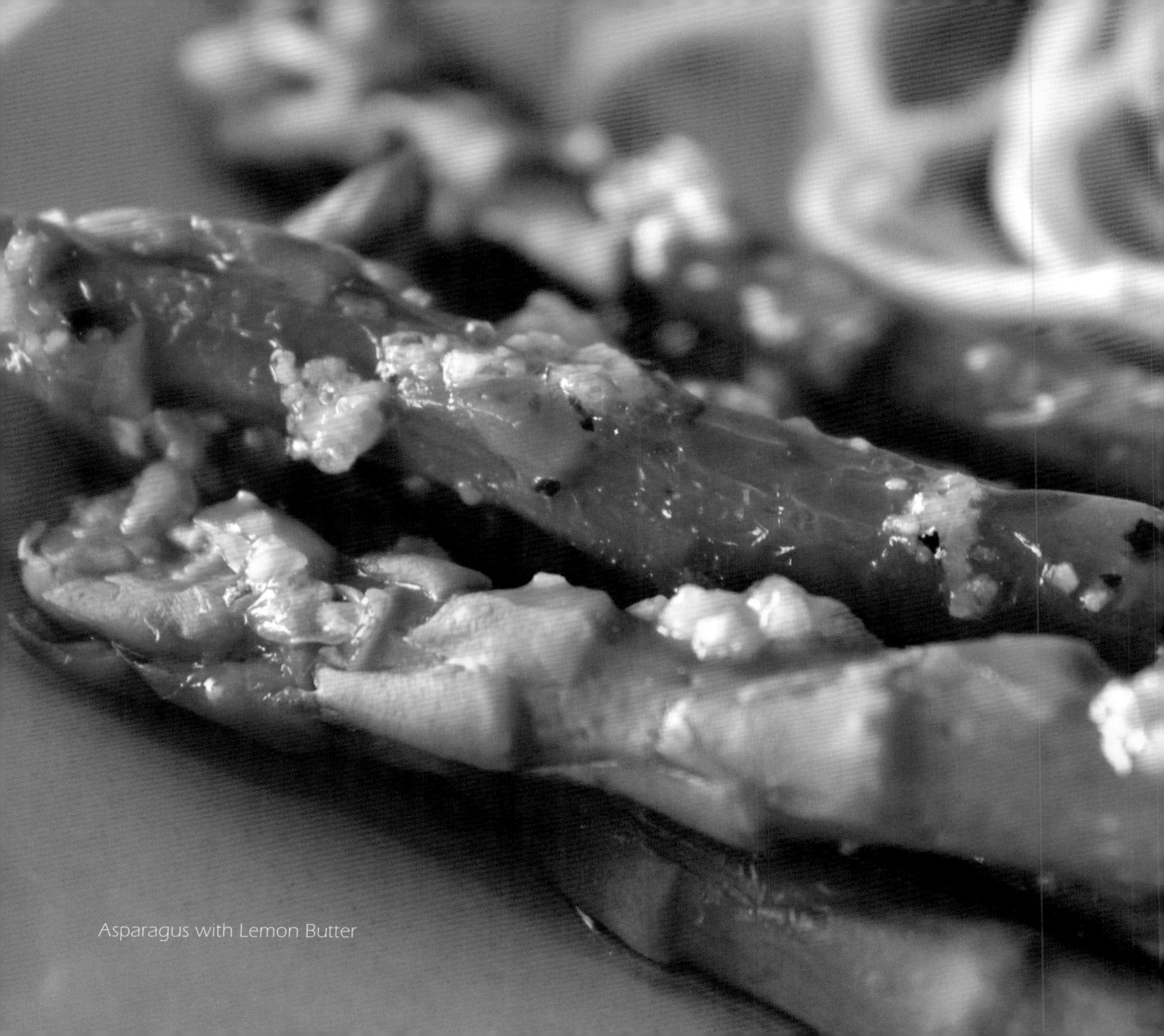

Asparagus with Lemon Butter

Asparagus with Lemon Butter

- 5–8 **asparagus stems**, trimmed
- 1 Tbsp. butter, melted
- 1 tsp. lemon juice
- ¼ tsp. grated **lemon zest**
- ¼ tsp. lemon pepper
- dash of coarse salt

1. Fill a medium saucepan half full of water. Bring to a boil. Add trimmed asparagus and cook for 6–8 minutes, until tender.
2. In a small bowl, combine butter, lemon juice and zest, lemon pepper, and salt to make lemon butter.
3. Drain asparagus and return to pan. Add most of the lemon butter and toss. Serve immediately and drizzle remaining lemon butter over asparagus.

Asparagus with Sweet Mustard

- 1 Tbsp. white wine vinegar
- 1 tsp. **stone-ground mustard**
- 1 tsp. brown sugar
- pinch of cinnamon
- 5–8 **asparagus stems**, trimmed

1. In a small saucepan, combine white wine vinegar, mustard, brown sugar, and cinnamon. Bring to a boil. Remove from heat.
2. Heat grill to medium-high. Add asparagus to grill and cook for 5–7 minutes, until tender.
3. Transfer asparagus to a plate and drizzle with vinegar mixture.

Parmesan Asparagus

- 1 Tbsp. **Parmesan cheese**, grated
- 1 tsp. garlic salt
- 5–8 **asparagus stems**, trimmed
- 1 Tbsp. butter, melted

1. Preheat oven to 450 degrees. Combine Parmesan cheese and garlic salt in a small Ziploc bag. Add trimmed asparagus and toss.
2. Place seasoned asparagus on a baking sheet. Drizzle with butter and remaining Parmesan mixture. Cook about 10 minutes, until tender.

Brussels Sprouts with Bacon

- 1 slice **bacon**, crumbled
- 5–7 **brussels sprouts**, halved
- 1 tsp. butter, melted
- 1 tsp. brown sugar
- 1 Tbsp. **pecans**
- 1 Tbsp. **dried cranberries**
- pinch of salt

1. Cook bacon in a small skillet until just barely crisp, about 2 minutes on each side. Remove bacon from heat and pat down with a paper towel to remove excess grease.
2. In the same skillet, add brussels sprouts, butter, and sugar. Mix well. Sauté over medium heat for 4–6 minutes, until brussels sprouts are tender and cooked through. (The thicker the brussels sprout, the longer it takes to cook all the way through.)
3. Mix in pecans, dried cranberries, and crumbled bacon. Let cool for 5 minutes.

Caramelized Brussels Sprouts

- 5–7 **brussels sprouts**, halved
- 1 Tbsp. unsalted butter
- ¼ cup **red onions**, chopped
- 1 tsp. garlic, minced
- 1 Tbsp. red wine vinegar
- 1 tsp. lemon juice
- dash of salt and pepper

1. Add brussels sprouts and ½ cup water to a medium skillet. Sauté over medium heat for 5–7 minutes, until most of the water is gone and the brussels sprouts are tender.
2. Add butter, onions, garlic, and vinegar. Cook for 5–7 minutes, until onions are golden brown. Add lemon juice, salt, and pepper. Mix well and let cool for 5 minutes.

Rosemary Roasted Brussels Sprouts

- 5–7 **brussels sprouts**
- 1 Tbsp. olive oil
- 1 Tbsp. fresh rosemary
- dash course salt and ground pepper

1. Turn broiler on. Cut brussels sprouts in half and spread out on baking sheet. Drizzle brussels sprouts with olive oil and season with rosemary, salt, and pepper. Broil brussels sprouts for 3–5 minutes.

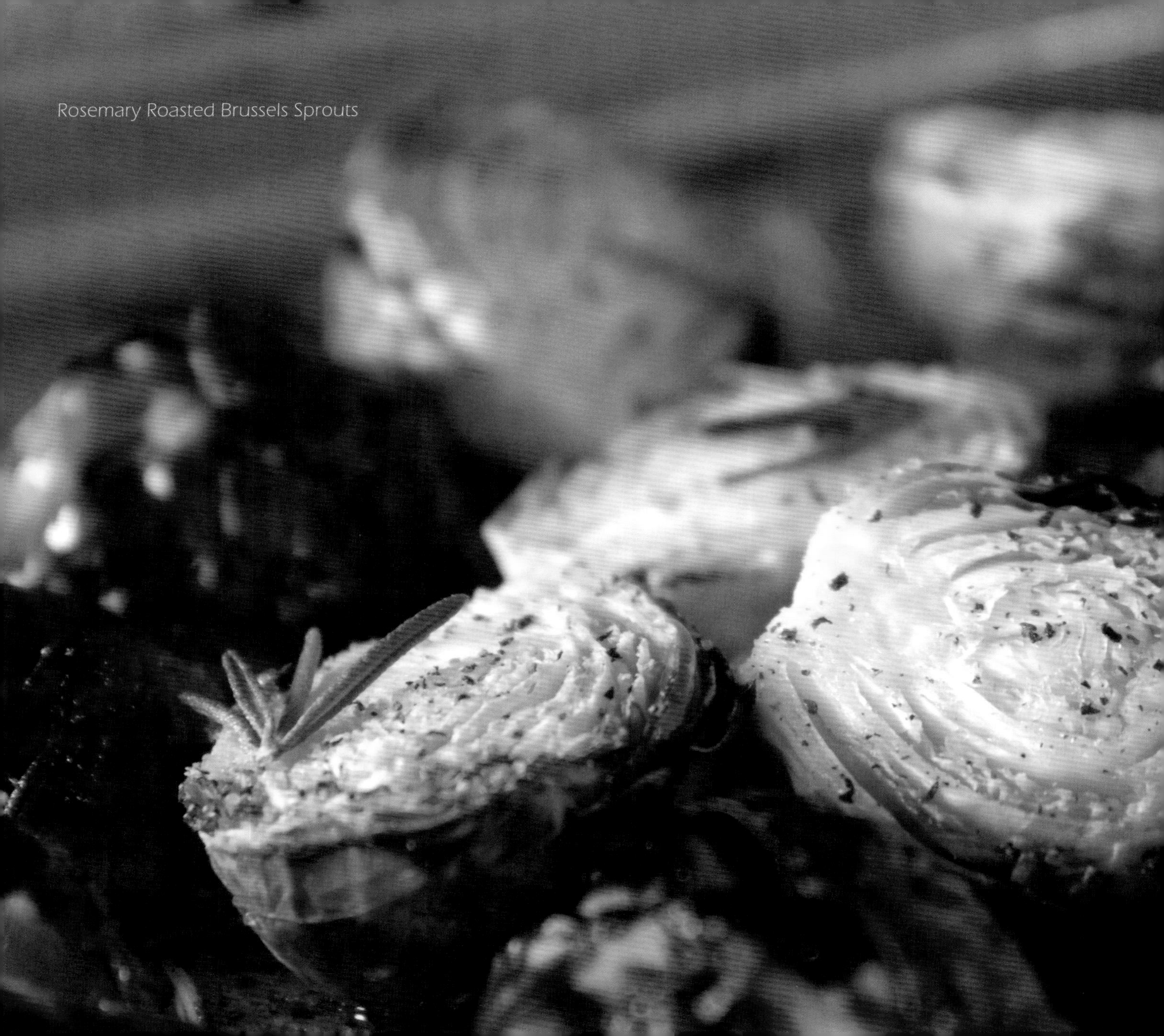
Rosemary Roasted Brussels Sprouts

Garlic Mashed Potatoes

- 1 large **red potato**, or three small red potatoes
- 2 Tbsp. milk
- 1 tsp. butter
- ¼ tsp. garlic salt
- dash of ground pepper
- ½ tsp. **Worcestershire sauce**
- 1 Tbsp. **cheddar cheese**, shredded
- 1 tsp. **fresh parsley**, chopped

1. Fill a medium saucepan ¾ full of water. Cover pot and bring water to a boil. Cut potatoes in fourths and add to boiling water. Cook covered for 15 minutes.
2. Drain potatoes and return to hot pot. Add milk, butter, garlic salt, pepper, Worcestershire sauce, and cheese to potatoes. Mash potatoes with a masher or mix with an electric mixer to the desired consistency. Add more milk, if desired, for a thinner consistency. Garnish with parsley.

Quartered Potatoes

- 3 small **red potatoes**
- 1 tsp. unsalted butter, melted
- 2 tsp. **fresh rosemary**, chopped
- dash of coarse salt and ground pepper

1. Preheat oven to 350 degrees. Cut potatoes in quarters, and place on a greased baking sheet. Drizzle butter and sprinkle rosemary and salt and pepper on top of potatoes.
2. Bake for 20 minutes. Let cool.

Garlic Basil Corn

- 1 cup **corn**
- 1 tsp. butter, melted
- ¼ tsp. garlic salt
- 1 tsp. **fresh basil**, chopped

1. Fill a small saucepan with water. Add corn and bring to a boil over medium-high heat. Let cook for 5 minutes.
2. In a small bowl, combine butter, garlic salt, and basil.
3. Drain corn and place in the bowl with the garlic mixture. Mix together.

Grilled Corn on the Cob

- 1 ear of corn
- 1 tsp. butter, melted
- 1 tsp. lemon juice
- ¼ tsp. coarse salt
- ¼ tsp. lemon pepper

1. Heat grill to medium-high heat. Remove husks from corn. Place corn on grill and cook for 15–20 minutes, turning occasionally to cook evenly.
2. Mix together butter and lemon juice in a bowl. With a brush, coat grilled corn with butter mixture. Sprinkle with salt and lemon pepper.

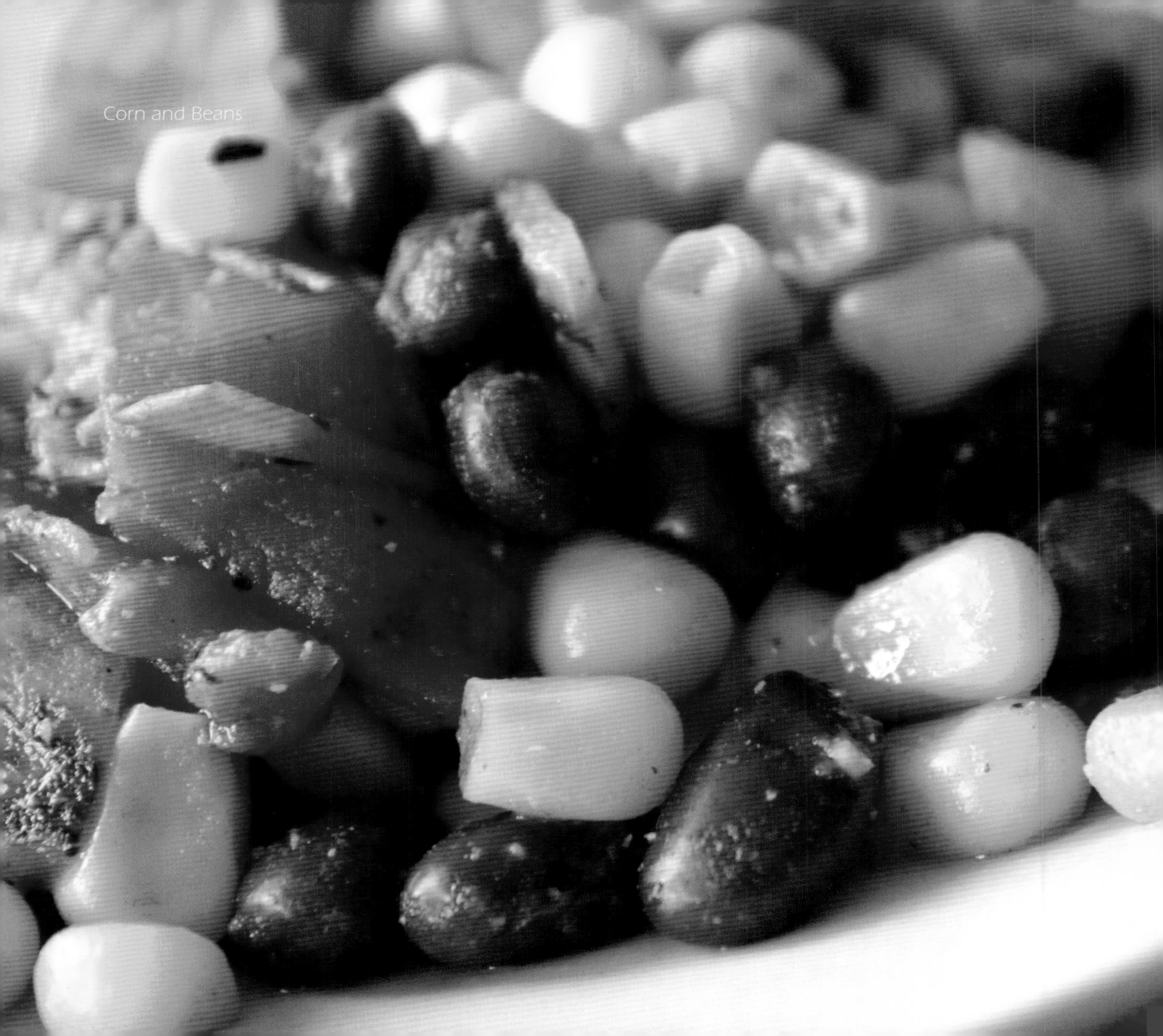

Corn and Beans

Corn and Beans

- 1 tsp. olive oil
- ¼ cup **red onion**, chopped
- ½ tsp. garlic, minced
- ¼ cup **corn**
- ¼ cup **black beans**, drained
- ¼ cup **tomatoes**, diced
- ¼ tsp. cumin
- dash of salt and pepper

1. Add olive oil, onions, and garlic to a medium skillet. Sauté for 5–7 minutes on medium-low, until onions are soft.
2. Add corn, beans, tomatoes, and 1 Tbsp. water. Cook for 5–10 minutes, until water is dissolved.
3. Add cumin, salt, and pepper. Mix well.

Black Bean and Tomato Quinoa

- ¼ cup quinoa
- ½ tsp. **lemon zest**
- ½ Tbsp. **lime juice**
- dash of salt and pepper
- ¼ tsp. sugar
- 1½ tsp. unsalted butter, melted
- ¼ cup **black beans**, rinsed and drained
- ¼ cup **corn**, drained
- ¼ cup **tomatoes**, diced
- ¼ cup **green onions**, sliced fine
- 1 Tbsp. **fresh basil**, chopped
- ¼ tsp. cardamom
- 1 tsp. olive oil

1. Fill a medium saucepan with water and a dash of salt. Bring to a boil over medium-high heat. Add quinoa and cook for 10 minutes. Drain and keep in sieve over a boiling pot of water for 10 minutes.
2. In a small bowl, add lemon zest and lime juice, sugar, salt and pepper, black beans, corn, tomatoes, green onion, basil, cardamom, and olive oil. Mix in quinoa.

Pine Nut Polenta

- 1 Tbsp. **pine nuts**
- ¾ cup water
- ¼ cup cornmeal
- ¼ tsp. salt
- 1 Tbsp. balsamic vinegar
- 2 tsp. butter
- 2 tsp. **fresh mint**, chopped

1. Place pine nuts on a greased baking sheet and broil for 1 minute, until golden brown.
2. Heat water on medium-high until boiling. Add cornmeal and remove from heat, constantly stirring. Add salt, balsamic vinegar, and butter. Stir until butter is completely melted and mixture begins to solidify. Add mint and pine nuts.

Roasted Tomatoes

- 4–6 **grape tomatoes**
- 1 tsp. olive oil
- 1 tsp. **fresh rosemary**
- dash of coarse salt and ground pepper

1. Preheat oven to 425 degrees. Cut tomatoes in half and lay with insides facing up on a baking sheet. Drizzle with olive oil, rosemary, and salt and pepper.
2. Bake for about 15 minutes, until soft.

Tomato, Basil, and Mozzarella

- 2–3 round **tomato** slices
- 2–3 round **mozzarella** slices
- 1 tsp. olive oil
- 1 Tbsp. **fresh basil**, chopped
- dash of coarse salt and ground pepper

1. Arrange tomato and mozzarella slices into a spread, alternating tomato and mozzarella slices. Drizzle with olive oil. Sprinkle with basil, salt, and pepper.

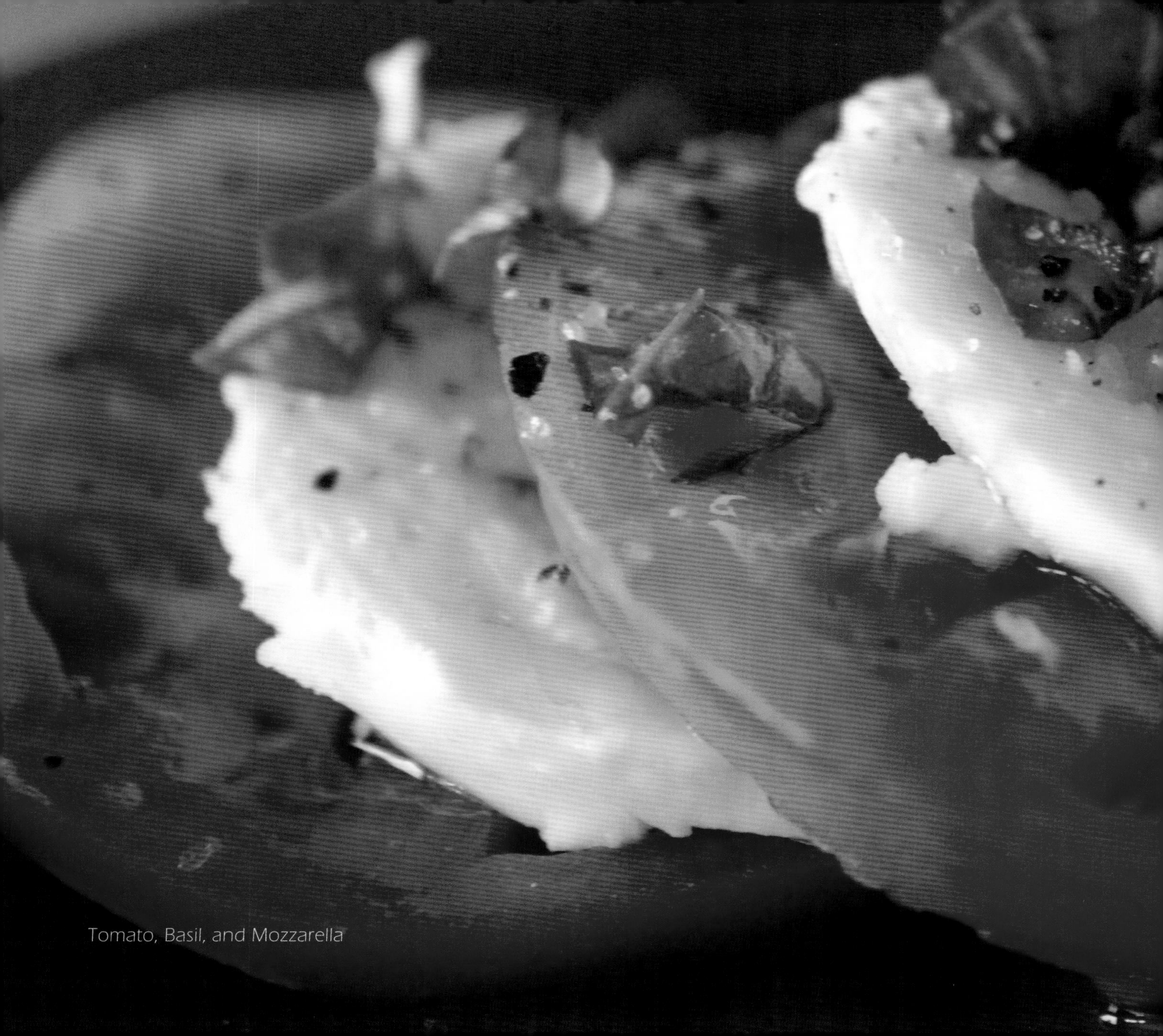

Tomato, Basil, and Mozzarella

Grilled Feta Tomatoes

- 1 medium **tomato**, sliced
- 1 tsp. olive oil
- 1 tsp. oregano
- 1 **kalamata olive**, finely chopped
- 2 Tbsp. **feta cheese**
- dash of coarse salt and ground pepper

1. Turn on grill to medium-high heat. Lay sliced tomatoes on grill and cook for 2–3 minutes on each side.
2. Remove from heat and place on a plate. Drizzle olive oil over tomatoes. Sprinkle with oregano, olives, feta cheese, salt, and pepper.

Sautéed Mushrooms

- 3 oz. **mushrooms**
- 1 tsp. lemon juice
- ½ tsp. **lemon zest**
- 1 tsp. white wine vinegar
- 1 ½ tsp. fresh oregano, chopped
- 1 Tbsp. extra-virgin olive oil

1. Slice each mushroom into quarters.
2. In a small bowl combine lemon, lemon zest, white wine vinegar, and oregano.
3. Heat olive oil in a small skillet. Add mushrooms and lemon mixture. Sauté for 5–7 minutes over medium heat, until mushrooms are softened, stirring occasionally.

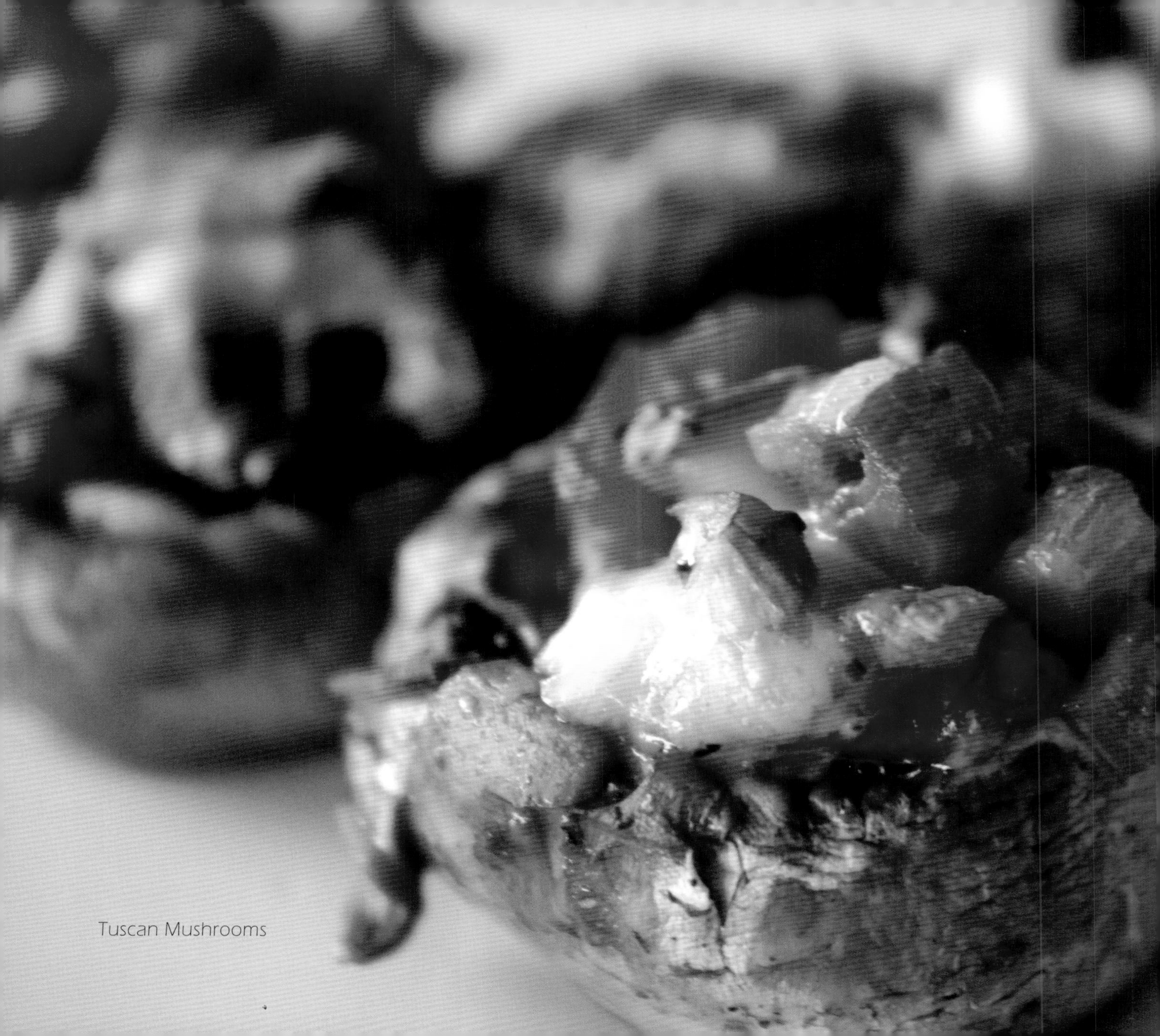

Tuscan Mushrooms

Tuscan Mushrooms

- 4–6 **white button mushrooms**
- 1 Tbsp. roasted red bell peppers, diced (from a jar)
- 1 Tbsp. pitted **kalamata olives**, diced
- 1 Tbsp. grated **Romano cheese**
- 1 tsp. **green onion** (white tips only), minced
- 1 tsp. olive oil
- pinch of salt and pepper
- 1 tsp. **fresh basil**, chopped

1. Preheat the oven to 400 degrees. Remove mushroom stems and dice them.
2. In a small bowl combine diced stems, bell peppers, olives, cheese, green onion, olive oil, and salt and pepper.
3. Place mushrooms on a baking sheet with the top of the mushroom facing down. Spoon mixture into the mushroom cavity. Bake for 10 minutes. Let cool. Garnish with basil.

Spanish Rice

- ½ Tbsp. olive oil
- ½ cup long-grain white rice
- ¼ cup **yellow onion**, chopped
- ½ tsp. garlic, minced
- 1 cup chicken broth
- ½ cup **stewed tomatoes**, with juice
- pinch of oregano
- ¼ tsp. salt
- ¼ cup **cheddar cheese**, shredded

1. Add olive oil and rice to a medium skillet. Cook over medium-high heat for about 3 minutes, or until rice is browned.
2. Add onion and garlic. Mix while cooking for about 3–5 minutes, until onion is tender.
3. In a saucepan over medium-high heat, add chicken broth and bring to a boil. Reduce heat to a simmer and add tomatoes, oregano, and salt. Mix well.
4. Add mixture from skillet to saucepan and bring to a boil. Reduce heat to a simmer. Cover and cook for 15–25 minutes (refer to instructions on the rice package).
5. Remove from heat and fluff with fork. Stir in cheese.

Wild Rice

- 1 cup chicken broth, divided
- 3 tsp. unsalted butter
- ¼ cup uncooked wild rice
- 2 Tbsp. **yellow onion**, chopped
- 2 Tbsp. **mushroom**, chopped
- 2 Tbsp. **almonds**, slivered
- 1 Tbsp. golden raisins
- pinch of salt and pepper
- 2 tsp. **fresh parsley**, minced

1. In a small saucepan, bring chicken broth and 1 tsp. butter to a boil. Add wild rice. Cover and simmer for 50–55 minutes, or until rice is tender.
2. Meanwhile, in a small skillet over medium-high heat, sauté onions, mushrooms, almonds, and raisins in 2 tsp. butter for about 5 minutes, until almonds are lightly browned and onions are tender.
3. In the saucepan, add almonds, raisins, salt, and pepper. Mix together. Transfer to a serving plate and garnish with parsley.

Apple-Butternut Squash

- 2–4 oz. **butternut squash**, cubed
- ½ **granny smith apple**
- ½ tsp. sugar
- ½ tsp. cinnamon
- 1 tsp. butter

1. Remove skin from squash. Cut into ½-inch cubes. Cut apple into ½-inch cubes. Add sugar, cinnamon, apple, and squash to a small Ziploc bag. Toss until fully coated.
2. In a small skillet over low heat, add butter, squash, apple, and extra seasoning from Ziploc bag. Sauté for 30 minutes, stirring frequently. After 15 minutes, add 1–2 Tbsp. water to keep moist if needed. Remove from heat.

Zucchini and Carrots

- 1 **zucchini**, sliced into rounds
- ½ cup **carrot**, grated
- 1 tsp. olive oil
- 1 tsp. garlic, minced
- 1 Tbsp. red wine vinegar
- dash of coarse salt and pepper
- 1 tsp. basil

1. Slice zucchini on a cutting board. Use a grater or a food processor to grate carrots.
2. In a medium skillet, add zucchini, carrot, olive oil, garlic, and vinegar. Sauté over medium heat for about 5 minutes, stirring frequently, until zucchini is tender.
3. Remove from heat and toss with salt, pepper, and basil.

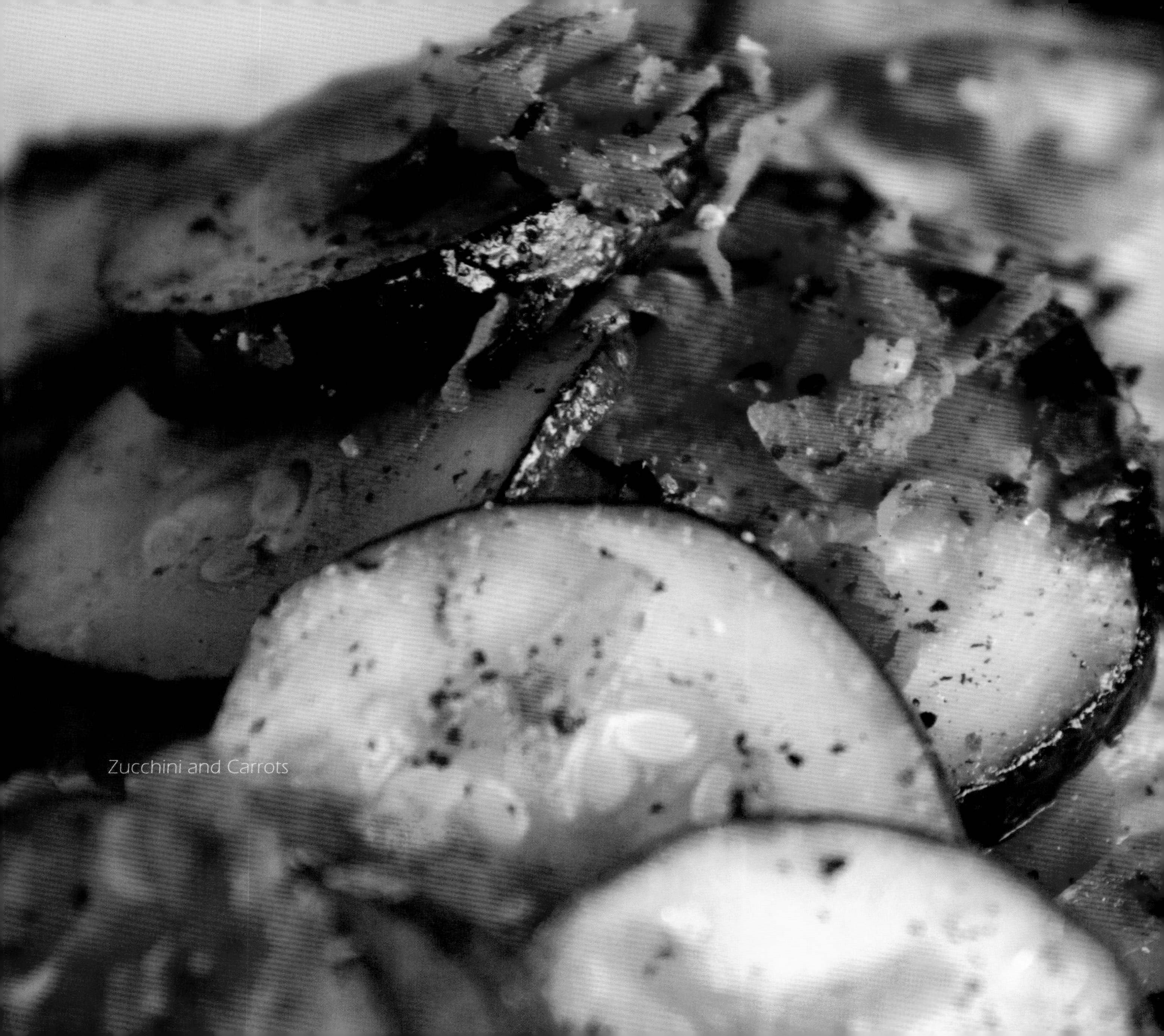

Zucchini and Carrots

Cubed Butternut Squash with Feta

- 2–4 oz. **butternut squash**, cubed
- 1 tsp. butter
- ¼ tsp. **fresh sage**, chopped
- dash of coarse salt and pepper
- 1 Tbsp. **feta cheese**

1. Remove skin from squash. Cut squash into ½-inch cubes. Add butter and squash to a small skillet. Sauté over low heat for 30 minutes, stirring frequently. After 15 minutes, add 1–2 Tbsp. water to keep moist, if needed.
2. Add sage, salt, and pepper to skillet and mix well. Let sit for one minute over heat. Remove from heat and toss with feta cheese.

Grilled Summer Squash

- 1 tsp. dill weed
- 1 Tbsp. white wine vinegar
- coarse salt and pepper
- 2–4 oz. **summer squash**
- 1 tsp. lemon juice

1. Add dill weed, white wine vinegar, salt, and pepper to a Ziploc bag. Shake and then add squash. Let marinate for 5 minutes, tossing frequently.
2. Heat grill to medium heat. Place squash on grill and cook for 10 minutes. Flip and then cook another 10 minutes. Garnish with lemon juice.

Maple Butternut Squash

- 1 cup water
- 2–4 oz. **butternut squash**
- 1 tsp. brown sugar
- 1 tsp. maple syrup
- 1 tsp. butter
- dash of coarse salt and pepper

1. Preheat the oven to 425 degrees. Pour water into a baking dish and then place squash in the pan. Texturize top of squash by running a fork across the top. Sprinkle the top with brown sugar. Cover with aluminum foil and bake for 45 minutes.
2. Remove squash from oven and scrape insides of squash from the skin into a small bowl. Add maple syrup and butter. Stir and mash well, until smooth. Add salt and pepper to taste.

Apricot Couscous

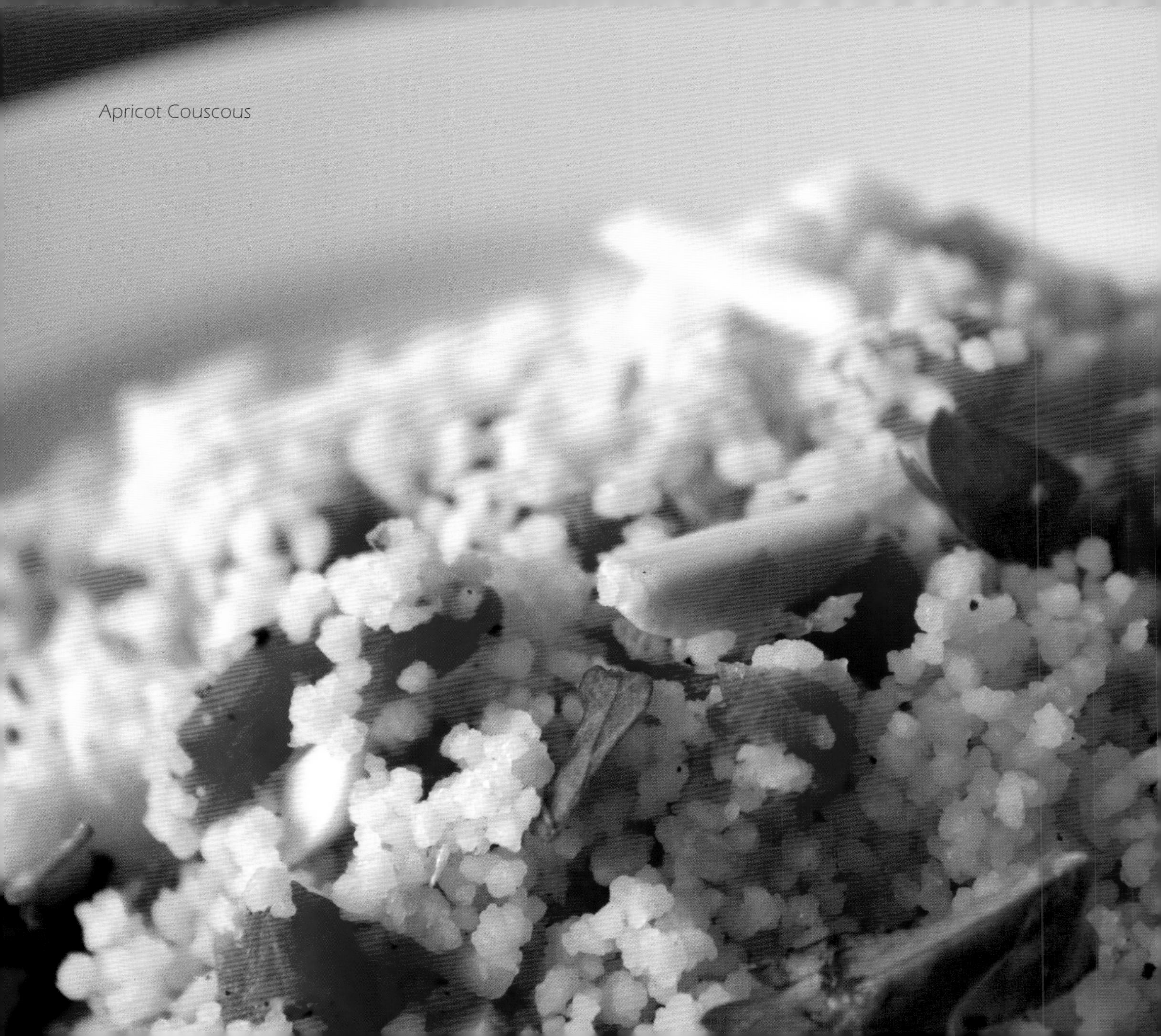

Mint Couscous

- ¼ cup **couscous**
- ½ cup chicken broth or water
- 2 Tbsp. **golden raisins**
- 1 Tbsp **pecans**, toasted
- 1 Tbsp. lemon juice
- 2 tsp. **fresh mint**, finely chopped
- dash of salt and pepper

1. Prepare couscous using chicken broth (or water) according to the package.
2. Fluff couscous with a fork and mix in raisins, pecans, lemon juice, and mint. Transfer to a plate.

Apricot Couscous

- ¼ cup **couscous**
- ½ cup chicken broth or water
- 3 **dried apricots**, chopped
- 1 Tbsp. **slivered almonds**
- ¼ tsp. **lemon zest**
- 1 tsp. lemon juice
- 1 Tbsp. **fresh cilantro**, chopped
- dash of salt and pepper

1. Prepare couscous using chicken broth (or water) according to the package.
2. Fluff couscous with a fork and mix in dried apricots, almonds, lemon zest, lemon juice, cilantro, salt, and pepper. Transfer to a plate.

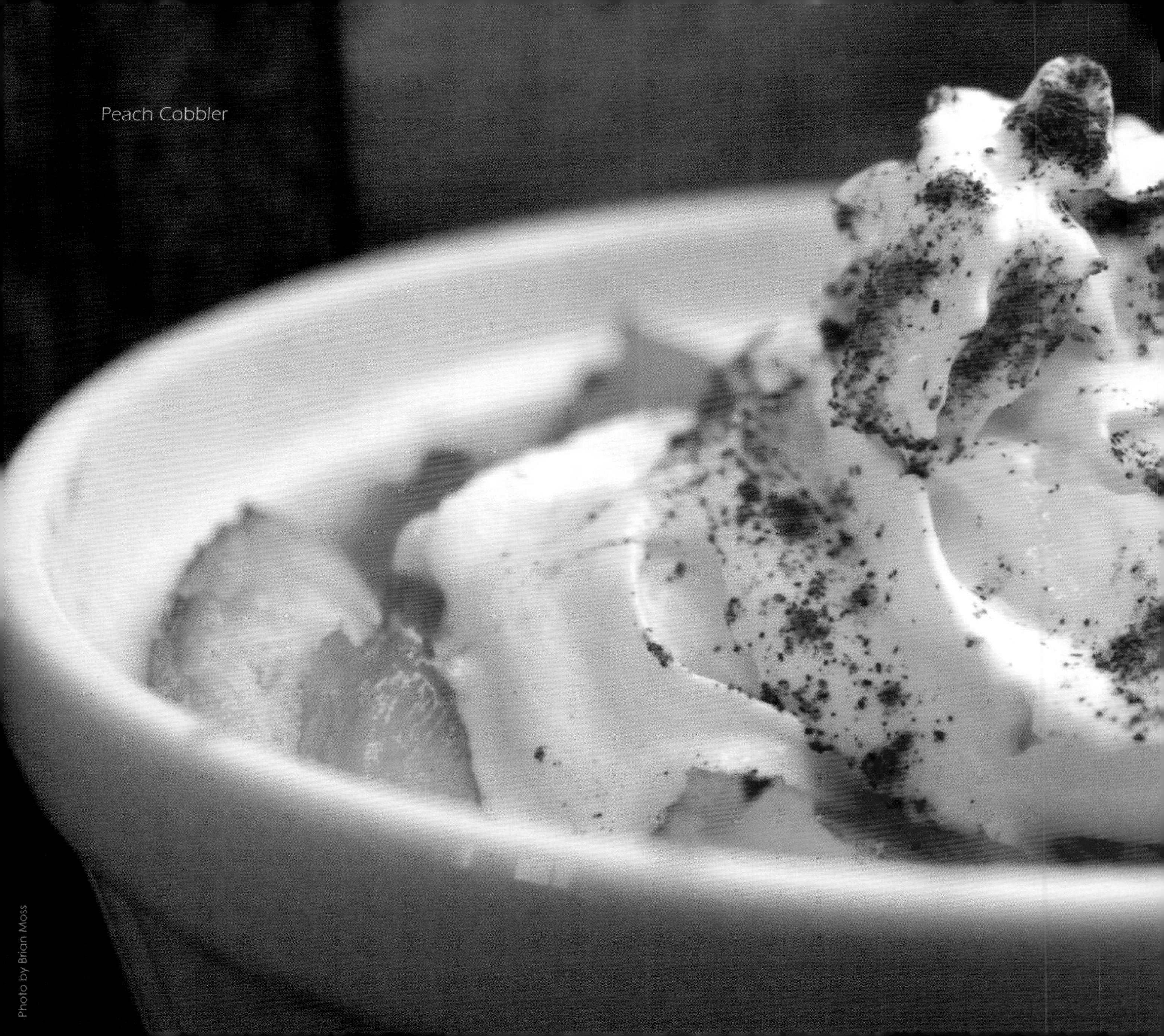

Peach Cobbler

Photo by Brian Moss

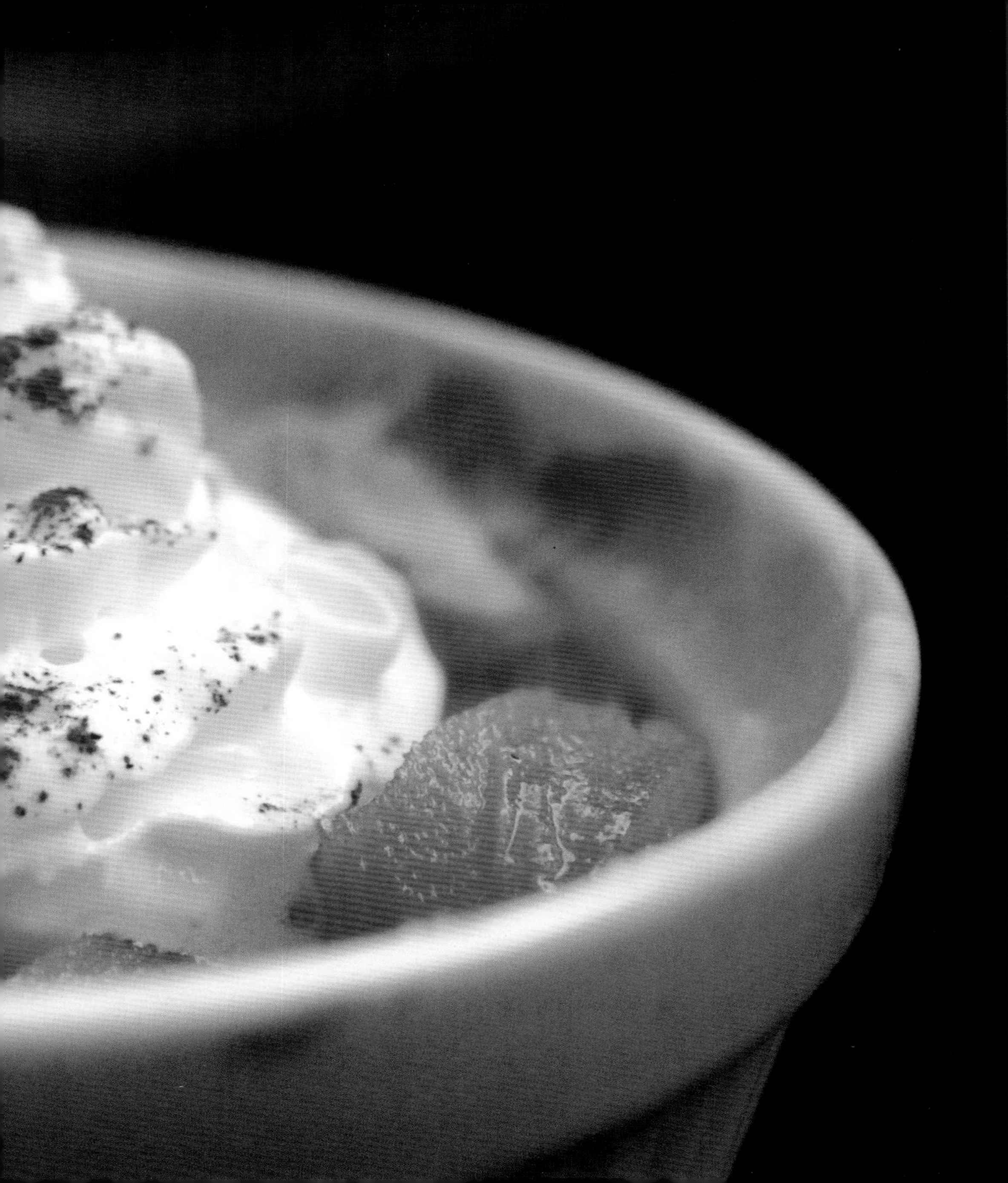

Dessert

Dessert

Dessert is probably the hardest thing to cook when you are single. It is quite rare to find a dessert recipe suited for one. While some might enjoy the extra dessert, others find that it only brings remorse. Let's face it; hardly anyone throws away their favorite dessert in excess, but instead consumes it over a couple of days. The problem is when you step on the scale, extra dessert usually converts to extra weight. For this reason, I've compiled some recipes that are scaled down to one serving, giving you a nice treat without the excess guilt.

Eggs

The first issue I had with some recipes was dealing with eggs. Typically, you size down a recipe to one egg, but in our case, I found a way to work around that. In several recipes you will see the instruction to whisk an egg and to pour in half, or another specific measurement (like 1 tsp.), into the dish. The reason for this is that eggs are essential in baking, yet the full egg distorts the reduced recipe. These directions will give you the right amount of egg to make the recipe taste just right.

Baking Dishes

Another issue I had with dessert was finding the right baking dishes. As mentioned previously, my favorite baking dish to use when cooking for one is the ramekin. You will see the ramekin used in three recipes: Chocolate Caramel Deluxe, Lemon Bars, and Peach Cobbler. Ramekins can be bought in all different sizes. I use ramekin dishes with diameters of 3 or 5 inches, which is specified in the recipes.

Healthy Substitutes

I liked to add fresh fruits to my desserts. Fruit has natural sweeteners, so you don't need to add much more to get the sweetness you crave. Additionally, several recipes in the cookbook call for fresh fruit, which helps you use the produce you purchase. However, for those recipes that don't have fruit, this list of healthy substitutes for common baking ingredients should help eliminate some calories.[1]

Baking Ingredient	Healthy Substitute
Butter	canola, mild olive oil, prune purée, or applesauce
1 ounce chocolate	3 tablespoons cocoa
2 eggs	2 egg whites or ¼ cup egg substitute
cream, whole milk	skim or low-fat (1%) milk
cream cheese (in cheesecake)	lowfat ricotta + yogurt; light cream cheese
sour cream	plain yogurt
whipped cream, ice cream (topping)	frozen yogurt, lowfat yogurt
1 cup whipping or heavy cream	1 cup evaporated skim milk cream
1 cup oil (in muffins, breads)	½ cup baby food fruit or vegetable + ½ cup oil or 1% buttermilk
evaporated whole milk	evaporated skim milk

1 Referenced www.globalgormet.com and www.cfs.purdue.edu.

Berry Parfait

- ½ cup granola
- ½ cup **vanilla yogurt**
- ¼ cup **raspberries**
- ¼ cup **blackberries**
- 2 tsp. honey

1. Layer the following (in order) in a small serving cup: ¼ cup granola, ¼ cup yogurt, 2 Tbsp. raspberries, 2 Tbsp. blackberries, 1 tsp. honey, ¼ cup granola, ¼ cup yogurt, 2 Tbsp. raspberries, 2 Tbsp. blackberries, 1 tsp. honey.

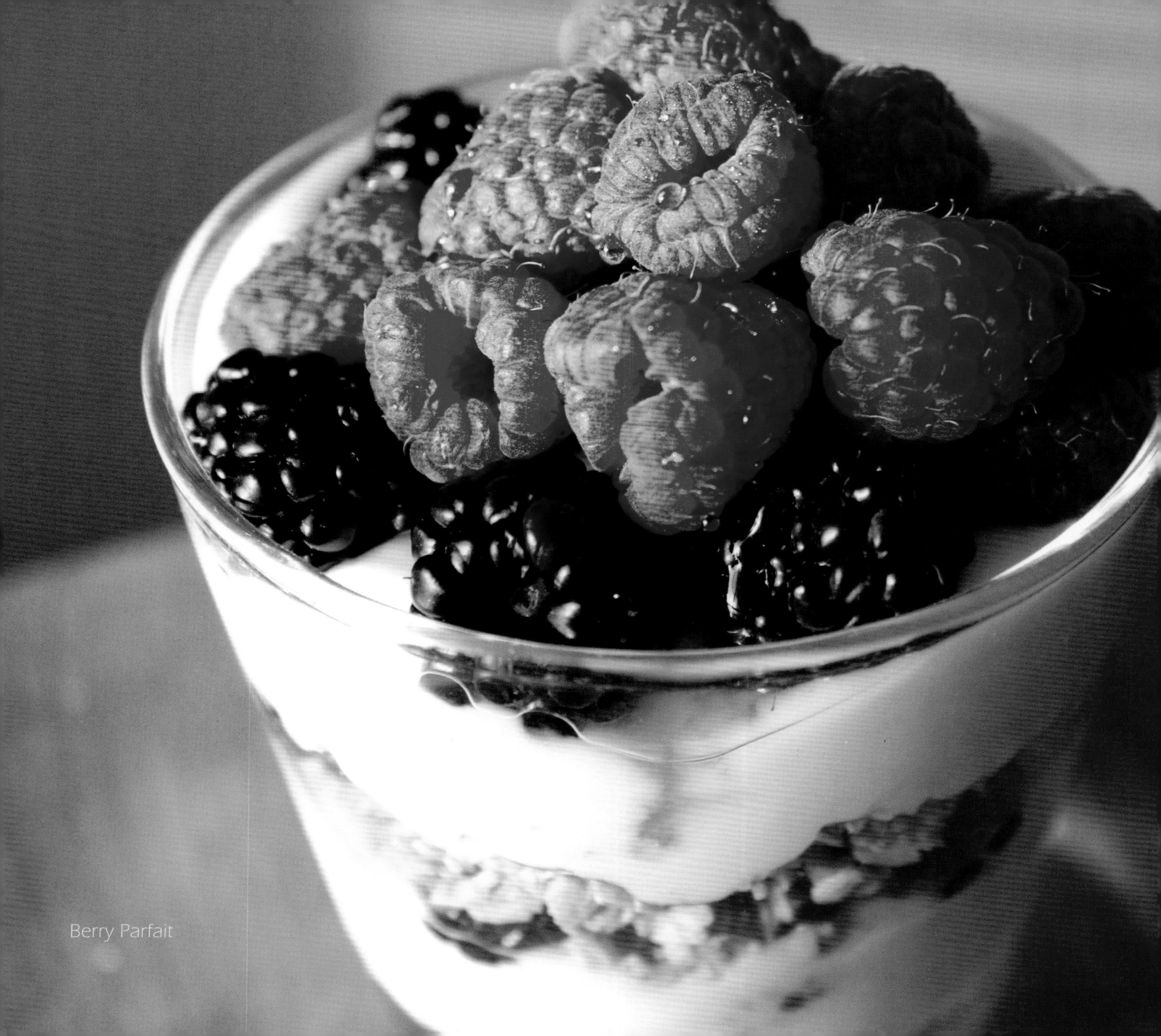

Berry Parfait

Apple Pie

Pastry dough

- ¾ cup flour
- ¼ tsp. salt
- 1½ tsp. sugar
- 6 Tbsp. unsalted butter, room temp.
- 1½ tsp. water
- 1 tsp. whisked egg

Apple mixture

- 1 **apple**, peeled, cored, and sliced
- 1½ Tbsp. sugar
- 1 tsp. flour
- 1/8 tsp. cinnamon
- 1½ tsp. lemon juice

1. Preheat oven to 375 degrees. Combine flour, salt, and sugar in a mixing bowl. Mix in butter, preferably in a food processor (15–20 pulses). Add ½ tsp. water and mix until dough is ready to knead. Put dough in refrigerator for half an hour to set.
2. Meanwhile, combine apple (of your choice), sugar, flour, cinnamon, and lemon juice in a small bowl.
3. Remove dough from refrigerator. Flour your surface and use a rolling pin to roll out the dough until it is ¼-inch thin. Use ¾ of the dough to place in bottom of a 5-inch ramekin.
4. Spoon in apple mixture. Cover with remaining dough and cut vents in dough cover.
5. In a small bowl, combine egg and 1 tsp. water. Brush top of dough with egg yolk mixture.
6. Place dish on baking sheet and bake for 35 minutes. Let cool for 5 minutes.

Butterscotch Pudding

- ¼ cup brown sugar
- 1 Tbsp. cornstarch
- dash of salt
- 1 egg yolk
- ½ cup whole milk
- ¼ cup **evaporated milk**
- 1½ tsp. unsalted butter
- ½ tsp. vanilla extract
- **whipped cream**
- dash of cinnamon

1. In a bowl, whisk together sugar, cornstarch, salt, and egg yolk. Add whole milk and whisk until light and fluffy.
2. Heat evaporated milk in microwave for about 2 minutes. Pour evaporated milk in a small saucepan and bring to a boil. Add egg mixture and whisk constantly for about 2 minutes, until mixture thickens.
3. Remove from heat and whisk in butter and vanilla extract. Pour into serving dish and let cool for 5 minutes. Garnish with whipped cream and a dash of cinnamon.

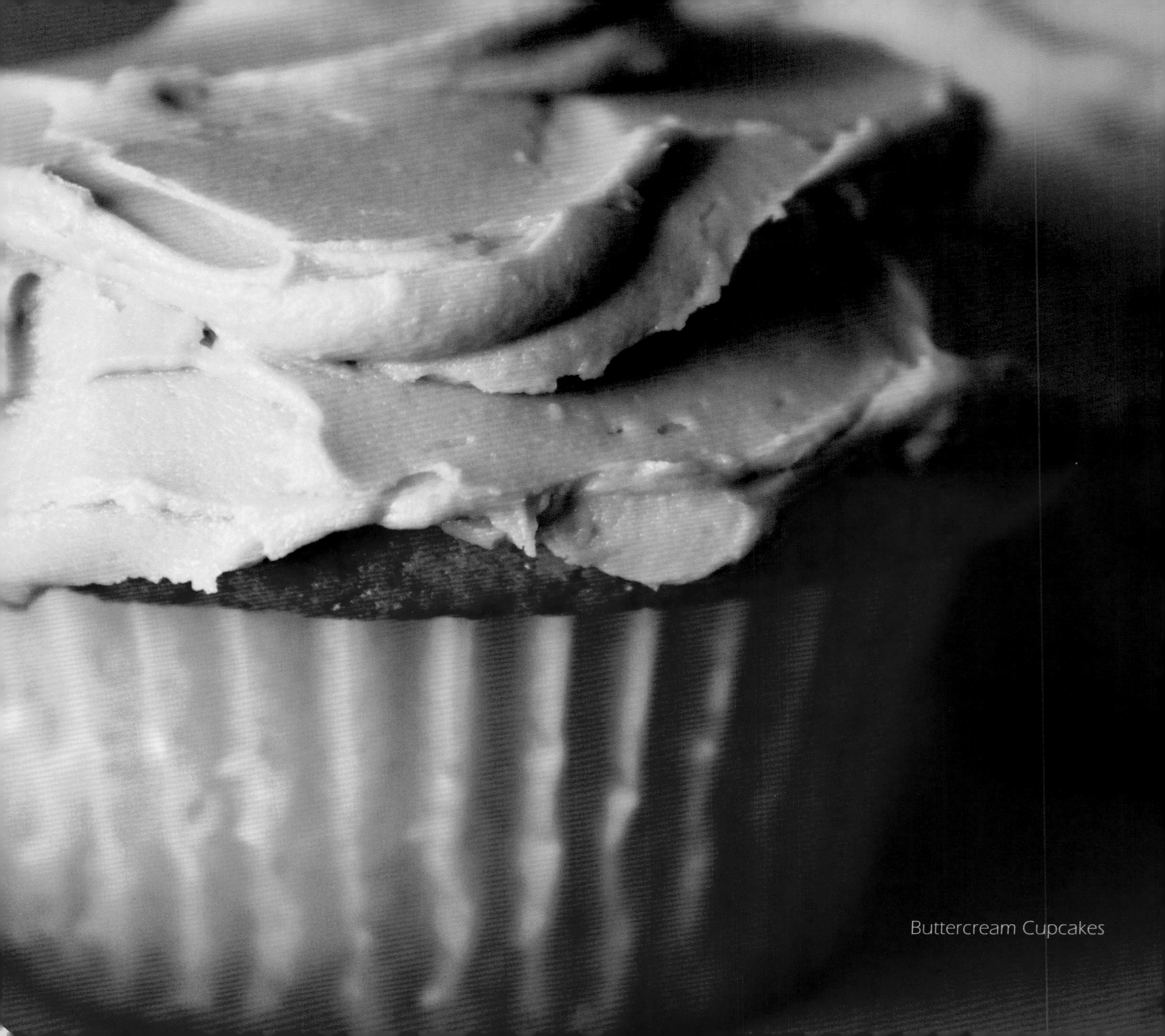

Buttercream Cupcakes

Buttercream Cupcakes

Cupcake

- 2 Tbsp. unsalted butter, softened
- 3 Tbsp. sugar
- ½ of a whisked egg
- 1/8 tsp. vanilla extract
- 1 ½ tsp. **heavy whipping cream** (or **milk**)
- ¼ cup flour, preferably cake flour
- 1/8 tsp. baking powder
- pinch of salt

Buttercream Frosting

- 2 Tbsp. unsalted butter, room temp.
- 1/3 cup powdered (confectioners') sugar
- 1/8 tsp. almond extract
- food coloring

1. Preheat oven to 350 degrees. In a bowl, mix butter and sugar, until light and fluffy. Add egg, vanilla, and whipping cream and mix well. Add flour, baking powder, and salt. Mix well.
2. In a cupcake pan, divvy out the batter into two cupcake holders. Place pan in oven and bake for about 22 minutes. Remove from oven and let cool for 10 minutes.
3. Meanwhile, make frosting by combining butter, powdered sugar, and almond extract. Add food coloring as desired. Frost cupcakes after they have cooled. Makes two cupcakes.

Carrot Cupcakes

Cupcake

- 2½ Tbsp. flour
- dash of baking soda
- dash of cinnamon
- dash of nutmeg
- dash of salt
- 2½ Tbsp. sugar
- 1½ tsp. whisked egg
- 2½ Tbsp. vegetable oil
- 1 tsp. **orange juice**
- 1/8 tsp. vanilla
- 2 Tbsp. **carrots**, shredded
- 1 Tbsp. **walnuts**, chopped

Cream Cheese Frosting

- ¼ cup **cream cheese**
- 1 Tbsp. unsalted butter, room temp.
- ¼ cup powdered (confectioners') sugar
- 1/8 tsp. vanilla

1. Preheat oven to 350 degrees. Mix together flour, baking soda, cinnamon, nutmeg, salt, and sugar. Add egg, oil, orange juice, vanilla, carrots, and walnuts. Mix well.
2. In a cupcake pan, divvy out the batter into two cupcake holders. Bake for 25 minutes. Remove from oven and let cool for 10 minutes.
3. Meanwhile, make frosting. Combine cream cheese, butter, powdered sugar, and vanilla. Frost cupcakes after they have cooled. Makes two cupcakes.

Cheesecake Sunday

- 1 Tbsp. **raspberry preserves**
- 1 Tbsp. **cream cheese**
- 2 scoops vanilla ice cream
- 1 graham cracker

1. Mix raspberry preserves and cream cheese in a small bowl. Heat for 15 seconds in the microwave to loosen up the mixture.
2. Add vanilla ice cream to a serving cup. Drizzle raspberry mixture over ice cream. Crumble graham cracker over the top.

Crêpes with Mixed Berries

Crêpes

- ⅓ cup milk
- ¼ cup flour
- ½ egg, whisked
- ½ tsp. sugar
- pinch of salt
- ¾ tsp. unsalted butter, plus more for pan

Fruit

- ¼ cup **blueberries**
- ¼ cup **raspberries**
- ¼ cup **blackberries**
- 1 Tbsp. sugar (or **vanilla yogurt**)
- dash of powdered (confectioners') sugar
- 1 Tbsp. **raspberry preserves**

1. In a small bowl, make crêpe batter by mixing together milk, flour, egg, sugar, salt, and butter.
2. Heat a medium nonstick skillet over medium-high heat. Dip a folded paper towel into extra melted butter; wipe bottom of skillet with buttered towel before each crêpe is poured. Pour ¼ cup batter into skillet; swirl skillet so batter coats bottom with a thin, even layer. Cook for about 1 minute, until edges are dry.
3. Using a spatula, gently lift one edge of crêpe, and flip the crêpe over; cook for 30 seconds. Slide cooked crêpe out of skillet onto plate. Repeat with remaining batter (batter will make 2–3 crêpes).
4. In a medium bowl, combine blueberries, raspberries, and blackberries with sugar (or yogurt). Place a few spoonfuls of mixed fruit in each crêpe and wrap taco style. Garnish with powdered sugar and warmed raspberry preserves.

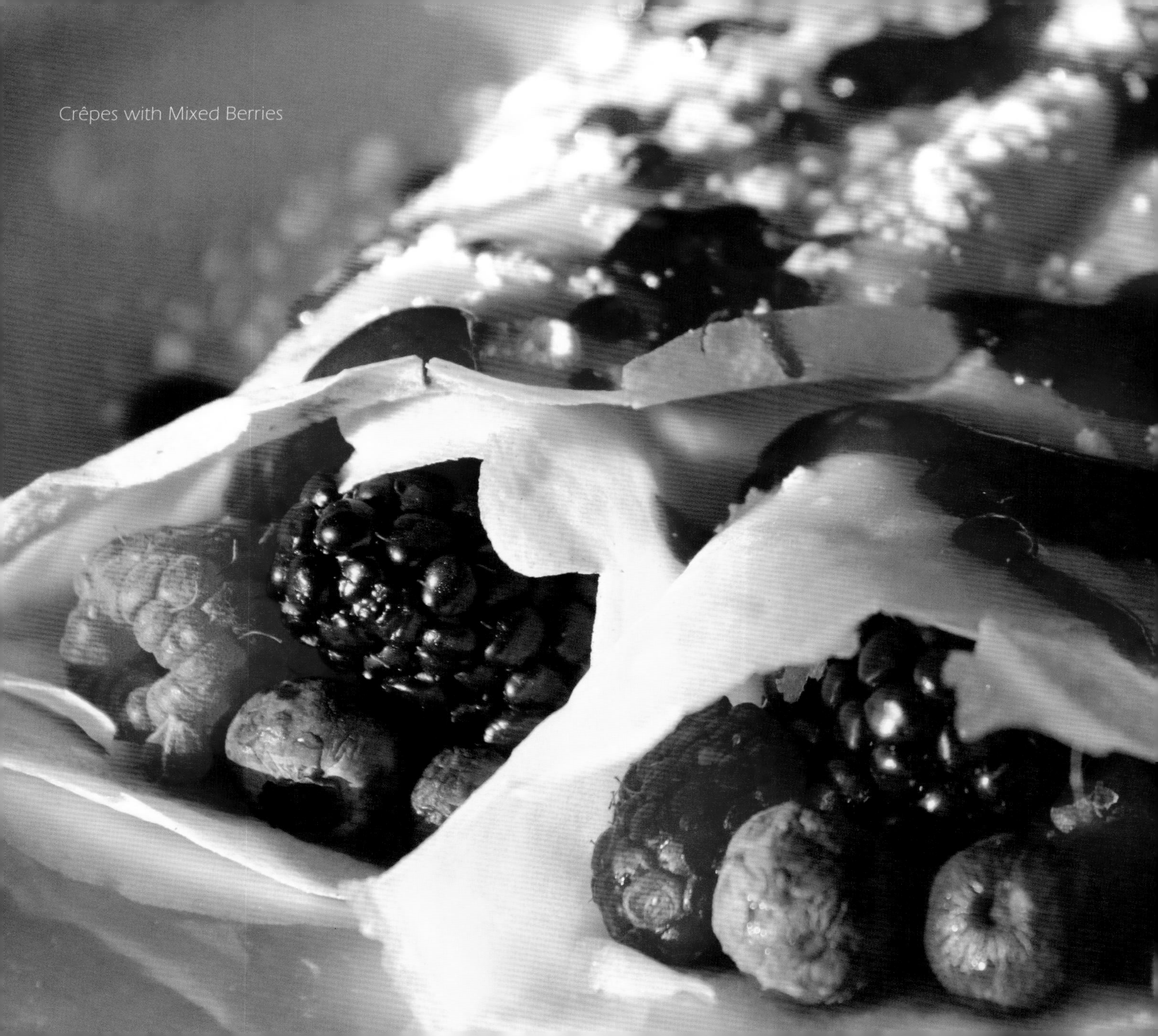
Crêpes with Mixed Berries

Chocolate Chip Cookies

- 3 Tbsp. unsalted butter, softened
- ¼ cup brown sugar
- 2 Tbsp. sugar
- 1/8 tsp. vanilla
- pinch of salt
- 1 egg yolk
- ½ cup flour
- pinch of baking soda
- 1/3 oz. **milk chocolate chips**

1. Preheat oven to 325 degrees. In a medium bowl, add butter, brown sugar, sugar, vanilla, salt, and egg yolk. Mix thoroughly. Add flour and baking soda and mix well. Mix in chocolate chips.
2. Put wax paper on a baking sheet (or grease a baking sheet). Fill a ¼ measuring cup with dough and plop on baking sheet. With your fingers, press the mixture and open like a flower, making the dough double in circumference. Bake for 15–17 minutes. Let cool for about 5 minutes. Makes 3 cookies.

Chocolate Dipped Pretzels

- 1 oz. **white chocolate chips**
- 2 oz. **milk chocolate chips**
- 3–5 pretzel rods

1. Separate white and brown chocolate into two bowls. Microwave each bowl on high for about 1 minute. Remove from microwave and stir. Continue to heat in 15-second increments if chocolate is not completely melted.
2. Submerge pretzel rod in milk chocolate until half of pretzel rod is covered. Set on a baking sheet lined with wax paper. Drizzle white chocolate on top. Place in refrigerator for about 10 minutes to set.

Chocolate Strawberries

- 1 oz. **white chocolate chips**
- 2 oz. **milk chocolate chips**
- 5 fresh **strawberries**, whole

1. Separate white and brown chocolate into two separate bowls. Microwave each bowl on high for about 1 minute. Remove from microwave and stir. Continue to heat in 15-second increments if chocolate is not completely melted.
2. Dip each strawberry a little over halfway in milk chocolate. Set on a baking sheet lined with wax paper. Drizzle white chocolate on top. Place in fridge for about 10 minutes to set.

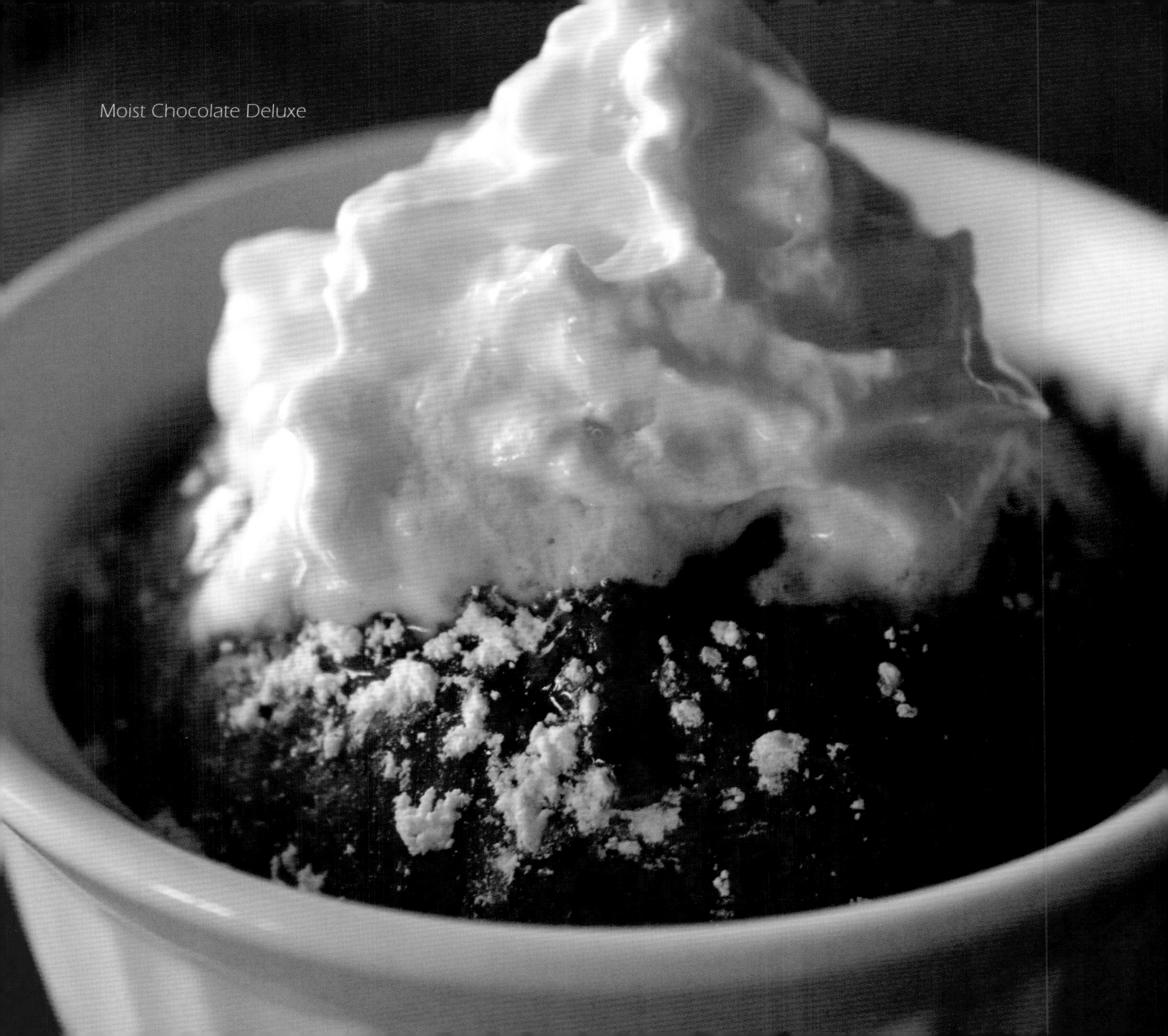

Moist Chocolate Deluxe

Moist Chocolate Deluxe

- 2 Tbsp. sugar
- 1 ½ tsp. cocoa
- ¼ cup flour
- dash of baking powder
- dash of baking soda
- pinch of salt
- 1 tsp. whisked egg
- 1 Tbsp. milk
- 1 tsp. vegetable oil
- ¼ tsp. vanilla extract
- 2 tsp. boiling water
- 2 tsp. **evaporated milk**
- 2 tsp. caramel topping
- **whipped cream**
- dash of powdered sugar

1. Preheat oven to 350 degrees. In a small bowl, mix together sugar, cocoa, flour, baking powder, baking soda, and salt. Add eggs, milk, oil, vanilla, and water. Mix well.
2. Pour batter into 5-inch ramekin. Place on baking sheet. Bake for 25–30 minutes.
3. Remove ramekin from oven and poke holes in the top of the cake. Pour evaporated milk and heated caramel over the top. Let cool to room temperature. Top with whipped cream and a dash of powdered sugar. Drizzle on extra caramel topping.

English Trifle

- 2 Tbsp. raspberry jam
- 1 cup sponge cake, cut in cubes
- 1 egg yolk
- 1 Tbsp. sugar
- ½ cup plus 2½ Tbsp. **heavy whipping cream**
- ¼ cup fresh **raspberries**
- 1 tsp. **almonds**, slivered

1. Spread raspberry jam on each cube of cake and place in bottom of serving cup.
2. Add ½ cup whipping cream to saucepan over medium heat and cook until scalding. Meanwhile, beat egg yolk and sugar in a small bowl. Pour egg mixture into saucepan and stir vigorously, until it is thick enough to coat the back of a metal spoon. Remove from heat and let cool.
3. Meanwhile, whip 2½ Tbsp. cream until soft peaks form. Spread cooled custard over sponge cake in a serving cup. Layer raspberries, whipped cream, and almonds on top.

Lemon Bar

- ¼ cup flour
- 2 Tbsp. powdered (confectioners') sugar
- 2 Tbsp. unsalted butter, melted
- 2 tsp. whisked egg
- ¼ cup sugar
- ¼ tsp. baking powder
- 2 tsp. flour
- 1 ½ Tbsp. lemon juice
- ½ tsp. **lemon zest**

1. Preheat oven to 350 degrees. In a small bowl, combine flour, powdered sugar, and butter. Press mixture into the bottom of a 3-inch ramekin. Bake for 15 minutes, until golden.
2. Meanwhile, in a small bowl, add egg, sugar, baking powder, flour, lemon juice, and lemon zest. Stir until there are no lumps.
3. Pour lemon mixture over hot crust and return to oven. Bake for 25 minutes. Let cool in refrigerator for 15 minutes. Sprinkle with powdered sugar.

Perfect Peach Smoothie

- ½ cup **plain yogurt**
- ¾ cup **apple juice**
- 2 Tbsp. sugar
- ¾ cup **peaches**, chopped
- ¼ cup banana, chopped

1. Combine ingredients in blender. Blend for about 30 seconds or until mixed thoroughly.

Summer Harvest Smoothie

- ½ cup **plain yogurt**
- ¾ cup **apple juice**
- 2 Tbsp. sugar
- ½ cup **strawberries**, chopped
- ½ cup **blueberries**

1. Combine ingredients in blender. Blend for about 30 seconds or until mixed thoroughly.

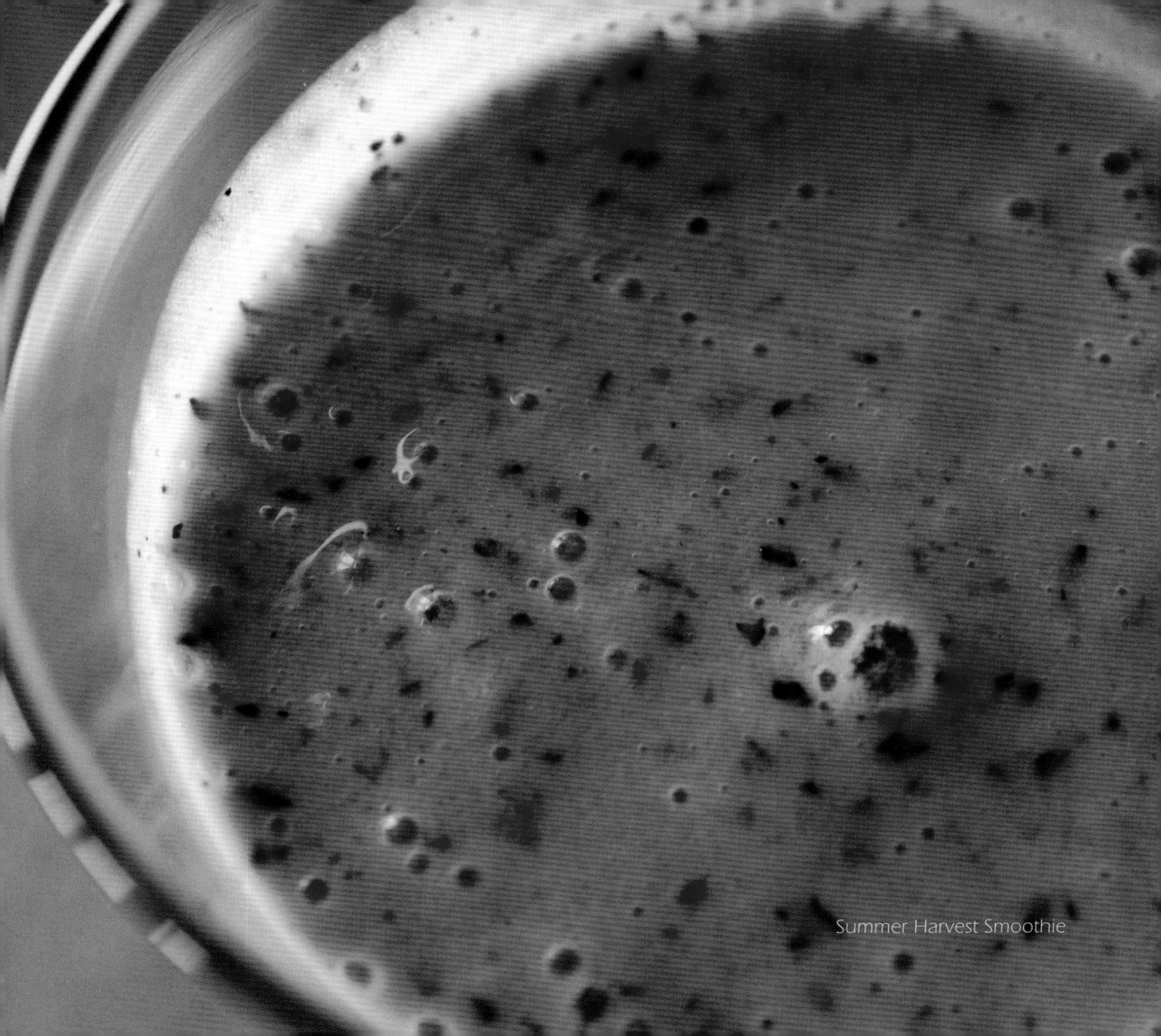

Summer Harvest Smoothie

Peach Cobbler

Cobbler Mixture

- ½ cup flour
- 3 Tbsp. sugar
- ½ tsp. baking powder
- ¼ tsp. baking soda
- dash of salt
- ¼ tsp. cinnamon
- dash of nutmeg
- 2 Tbsp. unsalted butter, cold
- 1/3 cup buttermilk
- **whipped cream**

Fruit Mixture

- 1 cup **peaches**, peeled and sliced
- ¼ cup sugar
- ½ tsp. lemon juice
- 2 Tbsp. water

1. Preheat oven to 400 degrees. In a small saucepan, bring peaches, sugar, lemon juice, and water to a boil. Let simmer for 10 minutes. Remove from heat.
2. In a food processor, combine flour, sugar, baking powder, baking soda, salt, cinnamon, and nutmeg. Add butter and pulse until mixture looks like small crumbs. Add buttermilk and pulse until mixture comes together.
3. Grease bottom of a 5-inch ramekin and spoon in cobbler mixture. Add peaches mixture and sprinkle with a dash of extra sugar.
4. Place in oven and bake for 50–60 minutes, until top is golden. Let cool for 5 minutes. Top with whipped cream and a dash of cinnamon.

Sugar Cookies

Cookie

- 1½ tsp. whisked egg
- ¼ tsp. vanilla
- 3 Tbsp. sugar
- 1¼ Tbsp. shortening
- 1¼ Tbsp. unsalted butter
- ¼ tsp. baking powder
- ½ cup flour

Frosting

- 1 cup powdered sugar
- ¼ tsp. vanilla
- 2–3 tsp. milk
- 1 tsp. unsalted butter, melted
- food coloring

1. Preheat oven to 375 degrees. In a medium bowl, combine egg, vanilla, sugar, shortening, and butter. Mix well. Add baking powder and flour.
2. Spread extra flour across countertop. Place dough on countertop and knead for about 1 minute. Using a rolling pin, roll the dough out flat. Use cookie cutters to cut out the shape of the cookies.
3. Place prepared cookie dough on greased baking sheet. Bake for 8–10 minutes.
4. Meanwhile, in a small bowl, mix together powdered sugar, vanilla, milk, and butter to create frosting. Add food coloring as desired.
5. Let cookies cool for about 10 minutes. Frost each cookie. Makes 3 cookies.

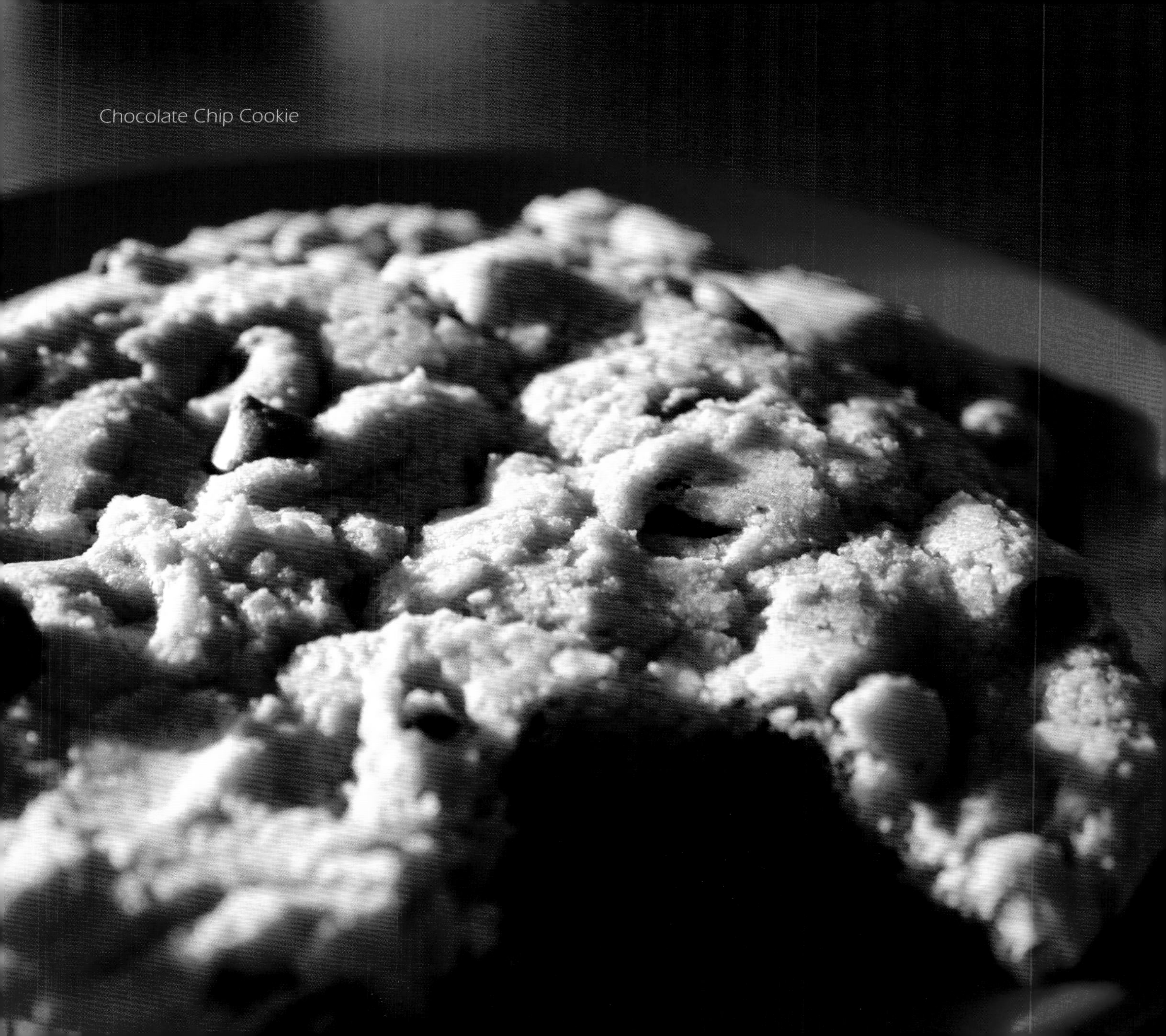
Chocolate Chip Cookie

Ingredient Index

Throughout this book you will see **bolded ingredients**. These are perishable ingredients that are common to more than one recipe. This ingredient index will help you find other recipes that call for the same ingredient to maximize your store purchase.

Alphabetical Index

Notes